The Business of
Nurse Management

Nancy Bateman, RN, BSN, is a Managing Director with Navigant's Healthcare Supply Chain and Clinical Redesign Practice in Phoenix, Arizona. Nancy specializes in clinical operations, supply chain operations, physician engagement, surgical services, emergency department and critical care redesign, and resource management. She is skilled in project planning and execution, team facilitation, communication, and change management. Nancy has successfully led process improvement, clinical redesign, and supply chain projects across the United States, Canada, and the United Kingdom.

Nancy has been a national speaker for National Nurses in Business, Healthcare Financial Management Association (HFMA), and World Congress and has been featured in several publications regarding her work, including *California Nursing Review* and *The Wall Street Journal*.

Nancy has more than 37 years experience as an RN and in health care consulting and operations, and 23 years concurrent perioperative experience. She has been certified in critical care, trauma, and operating room nursing. She founded and managed her own product research and development corporation in which she took several of her own product ideas from inception through the development, manufacturing, and marketing stages to the marketplace. Three of her ideas are patented.

The Business of Nurse Management

A Toolkit for Success

Nancy Bateman, RN, BSN

SPRINGER PUBLISHING COMPANY

NEW YORK

Springer Publishing Company, LLC
11 West 42nd Street
New York, NY 10036
www.springerpub.com

Acquisitions Editor: Allan Graubard
Senior Production Editor: Lindsay Claire
Composition: Absolute Service, Inc.

ISBN: 978-0-8261-5572-6
E-book ISBN: 978-0-8261-5573-3

12 13 14 15/ 5 4 3 2 1

The author and the publisher of this work have made every effort to use sources believed to be reliable to provide information that is accurate and compatible with the standards generally accepted at the time of publication. The author and the publisher shall not be liable for any special, consequential, or exemplary damages resulting, in whole or in part, from the readers' use of, or reliance on, the information contained in this book. The publisher has no responsibility for the persistence or accuracy of URLs for external or third party Internet websites referred to in this publication and does not guarantee that any content on such websites is, or will remain, accurate or appropriate.

Library of Congress Cataloging-in-Publication Data

Bateman, Nancy.
  The business of nurse management : a toolkit for success / Nancy Bateman.
      p. ; cm.
  Includes bibliographical references and index.
  ISBN 978-0-8261-5572-6 — ISBN 978-0-8261-5573-3 (e-book)
  I. Title.
  [DNLM: 1. Nurse Administrators. 2. Nursing Services—organization & administration. WY 105]
  LCclassification not assigned
  362.173—dc23
                    2011051117

Special discounts on bulk quantities of our books are available to corporations, professional associations, pharmaceutical companies, health care organizations, and other qualifying groups.

If you are interested in a custom book, including chapters from more than one of our titles, we can provide that service as well.

For details, please contact:
Special Sales Department, Springer Publishing Company, LLC
11 West 42nd Street, 15th Floor, New York, NY 10036-8002
Phone: 877-687-7476 or 212-431-4370
Fax: 212-941-7842
Email: sales@springerpub.com

Printed in the United States of America by Gasch Printing.

Contents

Contributors   *ix*
Foreword by Robert Doyle   *xi*
Preface   *xiii*
Acknowledgments   *xv*

PART I. MANAGING LABOR AND PRODUCTIVITY: THE NURSE MANAGER'S ROLE
Nancy Bateman

1. Understanding Productivity Measures   *3*
Nancy Bateman and Kara Allen
   The Relationship of Labor to Productivity   *3*
   Daily Staffing Plans   *7*
2. Staffing Models: Managing Capacity to Demand   *13*
Nancy Bateman
   Staffing Tools   *13*
   Applying the Flex Staffing Model to Labor and Productivity   *23*
3. Recruitment and Dismissals   *31*
Nancy Bateman
   Recruiting   *31*
   Importance of Performance Documentation and Reviews   *33*
   Performance Improvement Plans   *35*
   Dismissal of a Staff Member   *36*
Conclusion
Nancy Bateman

PART II. MANAGING NONLABOR AND SUPPLIES
Nancy Bateman and Thomas Behrens

4. Managing the Supply Chain   *45*
Nancy Bateman
   Nonlabor Expenses   *45*
   Supply Chain Spending   *46*
   What Are the Links in the Supply Chain?   *46*
   Managing the Supply Chain Budget   *51*
   Supply Costs and the Impact of New Technology   *53*

Financial Analysis and Cost Modeling   *55*
Value Analysis—A "Silver Bullet" for Supply Costs   *56*
Value Analysis Team Toolkit   *61*

5. Strategies for Achieving Cost Effectiveness   *69*
Nancy Bateman, Gregg Lambert, and Marilyn Connell
Group Purchasing Organizations   *70*
Supply Chain Contracting   *72*
Capital Equipment Expenditures   *76*
Inventory Management   *78*
Conclusion
Nancy Bateman and Marilyn Connell

PART III. FINANCE
Nancy Bateman and Pam Wright

6. Annual Budgeting and Purchasing as Part of Health Care Finance   *89*
Nancy Bateman and Pam Wright
Understanding Health Care Finance   *90*
Creating Annual Budgets   *95*
Purchasing Considerations From the Finance Side   *98*

7. Patient Care Reimbursement   *103*
Nancy Bateman and Anna Raneses
Centers for Medicare and Medicaid Services Reimbursement   *104*
The Process of Determining Illness Severity   *113*
Managed Care Contracts   *115*
Conclusion
Nancy Bateman and Jacklyn Mead

PART IV. RESOURCE MANAGEMENT
Nancy Bateman

8. Care Delivery Techniques for High Quality With Low Costs   *125*
Nancy Bateman
Resource Management   *125*
Determining Effective Patient Throughput Using Process Maps   *128*

9. Six Sigma   *151*
Nancy Bateman and Cynthia Tong
Six Sigma and Its Use in Health Care   *151*
Applying Six Sigma to Improving Health Care Outcomes   *154*
Conclusion
Nancy Bateman and Jacklyn Mead

PART V. DEVELOPING LEADERSHIP SKILLS
Nancy Bateman and Jacklyn Mead

10. Developing Personal Management Skills   **177**
Nancy Bateman and Jacklyn Mead
    Management Styles   **177**
    Troublesome Management Styles   **180**
    Team Motivation and Dynamics   **181**
    Communication   **187**
    Time Management   **194**
11. Skill Development for Managing Change, Conflicts, and Relationships   **197**
Nancy Bateman, Daniel Edwards, and Keith Hanchey
    Change Management   **198**
    Conflict Resolution   **203**
    Physician and Pharmacy Relationships   **204**
    Facilitated Sessions   **209**
Conclusion
Nancy Bateman and Jacklyn Mead

References   *219*
Appendix A: Helpful Websites   *221*
Appendix B: Sample Forms for VAT Toolkit   *225*
Index   *241*

Contributors

Kara Allen, MBA
Independent Consultant
Neenah, Wisconsin

Thomas Behrens, BS, MPM
Associate Director, Navigant Consulting
San Antonio, Texas

Marilyn Connell, BS
Managing Consultant, Navigant Consulting
Phoenix, Arizona

Robert Doyle, RN, BSN, MS
Managing Director and National Supply Chain
   Practice Leader, Navigant Consulting
New York, New York

Daniel Edwards, MBA, CRMP
Associate Director, Navigant Consulting
Houston, Texas

Keith Hanchey, BS
Managing Director, Navigant Consulting
Dallas, Texas

Gregg Lambert, BS, ME, MBA
Associate Director, Navigant Consulting
Nashville, Tennessee

Jacklyn Mead, BA
Educator, Writer, Editor
Avondale, Arizona

Anna Raneses, AAS, RYT
Vice President, Network Management, United Healthcare
Glendale, Arizona

Cynthia Tong, MSHA
Managing Consultant, Navigant Consulting
New York, New York

Pam Wright, BS
CFO, Cayenne Medical
Scottsdale, Arizona

Foreword

This book is an enthusiastic representation depicting the evolving role of our health care system's most valuable resource—the registered nurse. As health care in the United States continues implementing the Accountable Care Organization (ACO), we nurses must not only remain patient centric in the delivery of high-quality care, but must also become extremely knowledgeable about managing the "business of health care delivery." This book is meant to raise the bar on management techniques.

This work is more than a mere academic attempt to define basic management concepts, rather is a robust toolkit, providing real-life examples and experiences coupled with actual tools and techniques, allowing novice Nurse Managers to understand concepts such as supply chain management, financial management, and labor and productivity modeling. Additionally, this book serves as a roadmap to the successful implementation of these concepts. I think the author can be confident that there will be many grateful nurse leaders who will have gained a broader perspective of their evolving role and how to best implement those practices.

Robert Doyle, RN, BSN, MS
Managing Director, National Supply
Chain Practice Leader
Navigant Consulting

Preface

After 37 years in health care, I continue to see nurses promoted to Nurse Managers although they may lack the tools and techniques to support their roles. I began as a registered nurse and have progressed through numerous staff positions to become a clinical resource manager. I am now a managing director for a large global consulting firm where I work in the field of labor and productivity, nonlabor concerns, and clinical redesign. As a result of my experiences, this book provides advice and offers the actual tools and templates for nurses who are interested in managing staff and supplies effectively while promoting quality patient care.

Written with the help of several experienced colleagues, this book is a toolkit for newly promoted Nurse Managers, nursing students, and anyone looking to understand the business side of health care and to contribute to the viability of hospitals.

The information contained in this book is a result of the experiences assisting numerous clients across the United States, Canada, and the United Kingdom. Each experience with a client has added to the ability to incorporate new ideas and recommendations that have been included in this toolkit. It is this involvement and exposure to our clients' disparate issues that has brought about new techniques and enabled us to evaluate their effectiveness. Although each of our projects have involved similar challenges, each client has been unique and required adaptations to fit within its cultures and priorities. As a result, the tools and techniques offered in this book will need to be reviewed and adjusted to fit your needs. However, the book focuses on approaches that have worked well with the fewest revisions required across the experiences of the authors. The idea behind this book is to provide information on common issues to help readers see how their departmental needs fit into an overall operational picture.

The Bureau of Labor Statistics' *2008–2009 Occupational Outlook Handbook* states that nurses represent the largest health care occupation with 2.5 million jobs. Over the next 10 years, the need for nurses will increase by 587,000. There are 1,629 nursing programs in the United States today, divided as follows:

- 850 for associate degree programs
- 709 for bachelor and beyond programs
- 70 for other diploma programs

Many schools are offering RN to BSN and BSN bridge to PhD programs. These allow nurses with associates degrees (ADNs) to use employee education reimbursement programs to continue their education. As a result, many students choose to advance into a Nurse Manager position (Bureau of Labor Statistics, 2008).

Within this book, key elements of consideration for a Nurse Manager are discussed by chapter. Budgetary information, labor and staffing concerns, resource management, leadership skills, and supply management are delineated and discussed in great detail. I hope you find the book of value. Regardless of educational and vocational experience, this book can help any Nurse Manager gain new ideas and techniques for daily use.

Acknowledgments

This book was created from years of working with wonderful health care professionals across the United States, Canada, and the United Kingdom. As a consultant, you do not start by knowing everything; you learn from each professional you meet along the way. I loved working in surgical services, but after developing a latex allergy, I needed to look for another way to use my 23 years of experience in health care. Consulting gave me that opportunity. Every time I work with health care providers to reduce supply costs or improve care delivery, I incorporate all that I have learned from other projects. When the work is complete, I can then offer what I have learned to the professionals at the next project.

Along the way, I have broadened my knowledge because I was mentored by the best in the business. I am proud to have Robert Doyle as my mentor and author of the foreword for this book. Additionally, I thank John Walko and Dave Zito for all the years they kept me under their wings and taught me the business of project management and sales. All of the contributors are colleagues that have special skills and years of knowledge.

I thank my family for supporting me every day as I travel across the country and across "the Pond" every week to work. They have been especially supportive during these past months as I added the efforts of writing this book on top of the work schedule that often keeps me away from them.

Finally, I thank my daughter Jacklyn who has worked with me on the book, editing each chapter and acting as first reviewer.

The book is dedicated to my granddaughter Maggie. Her smile puts the world into perspective.

PART ONE

Managing Labor and Productivity: The Nurse Manager's Role

Nancy Bateman

The role and responsibilities of the Nurse Manager within the larger health care institution require a wide range of leadership and business skills. Successful management depends on the business acumen and experience of the manager who serves in a leadership capacity to inspire high-quality care. Application of business principles covered within these chapters will result in cost-effective delivery of services.

Understanding productivity and the various ways to measure progress will enable your department to continually improve. Delivering quality care under budget constraints can be accomplished with the appropriate care, proper delivery models, and use of daily staffing models that are flexible to demand. Components of a good staffing model incorporate departmental concerns as well as the acuity of admitted patients. Using these models to manage and measure labor and productivity within your department will result in recruiting the ideal candidates for employment. Finally, this section provides you with support for dealing with the removal of unproductive factors that may hinder quality performance. The case study at the end of Part I is a real-life example that illustrates the importance of the Nurse Manager's role within today's health care system.

Understanding Productivity Measures

Nancy Bateman and Kara Allen

The largest expense item within an annual budget is labor costs, including all professional, ancillary, and agency or temporary staff. Labor costs often represent as much as 60% of a Nurse Manager's annual budget. This chapter discusses the ways in which labor is monitored and measured for productivity. It also provides models and tools to build staffing grids, which can be used to track productivity in both bedded and nonbedded units.

Even the most educated and hard-working employees in your department may not be performing at their full potential. As a Nurse Manager, it is your responsibility to recognize where improvements can be made and initiate change. Being able to define productivity is essential to measure its progress. Understanding nursing ratios for all possible situations will provide you with the knowledge to manage daily staffing plans that effectively meet demand. A thorough understanding of productivity measures will allow all of your employees to thrive while providing the best quality care.

LEARNING OBJECTIVES

1. Define productivity and measure it.
2. Understand nursing ratios and how they impact staffing.
3. Manage daily staffing plans.

THE RELATIONSHIP OF LABOR TO PRODUCTIVITY

Productivity is often compared to specific units of measure such as "worked care hours" or "units of service" (i.e., emergency department [ED] visits). These measurements, however, do not account for nonquantifiable nursing skills, such as specialty skills and the provision of high-quality care at diminished costs. In other words, if professional nurses are caring for patients within appropriate ratios, they are likely providing the highest quality of care possible. But are these measures realistic and necessary? Just because there are professional nurses working in a department does not mean that their skills are matched appropriately to the type of patients being cared for. Nonclinical administrators often still believe that a "nurse is a nurse." When California first introduced the Title 22 statutes that mandated nursing ratios in 2004—a progressive move in relation to staffing and patient needs—many hospital administrators responded by reducing ancillary support to professional nurses. This action was an attempt to meet ratios without increasing labor budgets beyond affordability, although ratios were still difficult to meet, and labor budgets still grew.

The Advent of Ratios

The introduction of mandatory nurse ratios, when first launched in 2004 throughout California hospitals, was a progressive move toward assuring both staff and patients that enough direct professional care would be available based on unit type and patient acuity. Although the ratios were generally accepted, mandates associated with the ruling were challenged. Opponents to the ruling objected to the regulation requiring that all departments maintain ratios during breaks and lunches, requiring replacement nurses to relieve those on break. If a patient was in a critical care unit and was waiting for a bed to become available, the ratio would still be required. Administrative tracking of staffing records also needed to be held for a full year, with records including staff and patient names for each nurse by shift. In departments where patient flow was inconsistent, these records needed to be updated and filed hourly, and fast-track EDs were also required to maintain ratio figures. Table 1.1 outlines the ratios by department.

Many states have adapted variations of the California law. Two main issues regarding current regulations are the cost and the availability of professional nurses to fill all required positions. Cost issues resulted in many hospitals hiring more professional nurses (registered nurses [RNs] and licensed practical nurses [LPNs]). To offset the costs of the new staff, administrations laid off support staff and nonclinical staff, forcing nurses to care for a smaller number of patients while taking on the tasks commonly assigned to support staff. From an economic standpoint, this provided a poor return on investment because higher paid nurses were now performing low-skill tasks. For more information on resource management, see Part IV.

Productivity

Nurse Managers are responsible for the labor productivity of their department. In a hospital, labor productivity is a calculation of either worked hours or paid hours divided by a unit of measure reflecting the volume of work required in a unit. Both worked hours and paid hours are important things for a manager to understand and monitor. Worked hours include only those hours actually spent on a unit, typically including education and orientation hours. Managers are responsible for determining an appropriate number of staff per day for their unit. Paid hours include all worked hours plus any vacation, sick, and holiday hours. When staff members request vacation time, per-hour figures will increase as employees on paid vacation are compensated along with the substituted staff covering their absence. Keeping detailed records for worked hours and paid hours can help explain cost concerns with hospital administrators.

TABLE 1.1
Mandatory Nurse Ratios in California Hospitals by Department

Unit	Nurse to Patient Ratio
Critical Care, including newborn	1:2
OR	1:1, circulator
Pediatrics	1:4
PACU	1:2
Emergency	1:4
Emergency critical patients	1:2
Emergency trauma patients	1:1
Labor and delivery active labor	1:2
Antepartum, not in active labor	1:4
Postpartum mothers only	1:6
Nursery	1:8
Postpartum mother/baby	1:4 couplet
LDRP	1:3, 1 labor, 1 mom, 1 baby
Progressive care/ICU step down	1:4 till 2008 then 1:3
Telemetry	1:5 till 2008 then 1:4
Medical/surgical	1:5 assuming 2005 rule stands
Specialty units	1:5 till 2008 then 1:4
Psychiatry	1:6 includes LPTs like LPNs

Note: ICU, intensive care unit; LDRP, labor, delivery, recovery, and postpartum; LPNs, licensed practical nurses; LPTs, licensed physical therapists; OR, operating room; PACU, post-anesthesia care unit. Adapted from Title 22 California Code of Regulations, Section 70217.

The second component of the labor productivity metric is the volume number. The volume of work performed in a nursing unit is measured using a metric that correlates to the work of the department. For example, an OR will use a metric of performed surgeries, although an inpatient bedded unit will calculate their metric in patient days. Nurse Managers can control workload volume by instituting efficient processes because this permits additional flow without requiring additional staff. For example, a manager of an OR can locate high-use supply items in each operating room and lower the amount of time required retrieving them. This, therefore, shortens the length of the case, freeing the room for another case more quickly. Although it is possible to affect the efficiency of a department, there are many elements impacting volume that cannot be controlled: the availability of specialists and physicians, the movement of patients from other departments, and the hospital census are all examples of factors that can impact a department's volume and efficiency. It is important to be aware of these possibilities, keeping organized and ready for anything a department might face.

Conversely, it is also important to realize how one's department impacts the efficiency of other departments. A classic example of this is the amount of time required to ready a patient for transport from a bedded unit to an ancillary department. If a patient is not ready to be transported or if there is no one available to transport the patient, this can create a backlog that reduces efficiency.

After understanding the components of productivity measurements, it is useful to discuss a Nurse Manager's responsibilities and his or her ability to manage these measurements. The number of working staff and work volume within a department can affect productivity, requiring managers to set flexible yet reliable schedules. Nurse Managers should establish daily schedules because they can allow units to care for average patient census totals. Because census tallies change daily, it may be necessary to flex one's staff to match departmental volume. When a census is lower than average, staff can be sent to another department that requires additional support or can be sent home. If the census is higher than normal, additional staff must be called in to support the additional number of patients. Hospitals may fill additional staffing needs by making use of the following:

- **Float pool**—A group of nurses that are centrally managed, typically by the nurse staffing office. This is a group of trained nurses that are not assigned to any particular unit but rotate (or float) to units as needed. The hours a float nurse spends in a department will show up in a department's worked- and paid-hour figures. The rate of pay for float staff is the regular hourly rate and is therefore the cheapest method of supplementing staff, though there may be a slight learning curve for the nurse as he or she becomes acquainted with a unit's idiosyncrasies.

- **Overtime**—Overtime staff are asked to work additional hours on top of regularly scheduled hours. The rate of pay for this time can range from a time-and-a-half to two times the hourly rate depending on hospital policy, making the use of these employees more expensive than the use of a float pool. The advantage of using overtime staff is their familiarity with unit's processes and operations. Overtime staff provides a short-term solution but can cause burnout in the long term if used too often. The national benchmark for overtime is 2% of total labor expense. If overtime expenses exceed this amount, it will be important to review staffing plans and processes. The case study at the end of this chapter offers a real-life example of how changing staffing models can reduce overtime to benchmark levels.

- **Agency nurses**—Agency nurses provide the advantage of not overburdening staff. The rate of pay for an agency nurse is significantly higher than either overtime or float staff. If agency nurses are used extensively, it is worth reviewing staffing policies and adding full-time nurses because they are more cost effective.

- **Traveling nurses**—Similar to agency nurses, traveling nurses are supplemental staff provided by outside agencies. In contrast to typical agency nurses who are brought in for short-term work (a day or longer), traveling nurses are contracted for several months. Additionally, the rate of pay for traveling nurses is significantly higher than that of hospital staff. Traveling nurses provide staffing solutions for short, foreseeable deficiencies and are best used in instances in which new staff has been hired but cannot begin working for a short period. However, considering the added costs of these staff, it is important to reevaluate permanent staffing figures if traveling nurses are used frequently. Another disadvantage of traveling nurses is that a department must pay their contracted salary even if a census is low and other nurses are sent home during lulls in activity.

Another budgeting consideration not often addressed is the hours allocated from other departments. When other departments send staff to different floors, the hours spent may be allocated to that floor's budget. Attention must be paid to these hours so that corrective action can be taken quickly.

Common Terminology

To manage staffing effectively, there are many common financial terms that may appear within a health care setting that should be used by Nursing Managers. Table 1.2 provides many of these terms and the formulas for how to calculate them.

When considering your department's productivity remember that even though nursing ratios may be difficult to meet, it is worth the effort. Labor and productivity will still grow if you make sure you are staffing to meet demand. Track staffing records for one year to maintain ratio figures, monitor trends, and foresee possible complications. Knowing your ratios by department and any variations by state will keep your floor up-to-date. Being familiar with the common financial terms that pertain to health care will also accelerate improvements. Keep in mind that the efficiency of your department will also affect other departments within your hospital.

DAILY STAFFING PLANS

Managing daily staffing plans is an important component of maintaining productivity in your department. Although staffing grids are described in Chapter 2, managing these on a day-to-day basis requires attention to your daily census and to your patient population acuity. The challenge is in creating staffing plans at least two weeks out in order to post the schedule for your staff, while staying in budget because that relates to your department's productivity targets.

The two main areas to stay focused on are your worked hours per patient day (WHPPD) and your amount of overtime.

Each department—depending on the type of care delivered—is measured by units of service. As noted earlier in Table 1.2, your targeted WHPPD should be in alignment with benchmarked data and within your facility's expected quartile. Most hospitals subscribe to external benchmarking databases so they can compare their performance to peers. Each department uses different units of service and, as a Nurse Manager, you will be asked to set your targets for productivity. Examples of units of service are patient days for medical and surgical floors often referred to as a "bedded unit" because the patient is assigned to a bed. A nonbedded unit would be a department, such as the ED, where a patient is lying on a gurney and the service unit of measure is the number of ED visits. Departments that do not deliver patient care, such as materials management, are usually benchmarked with adjusted discharges for their units of service.

Once your unit of service is identified, then you compare your data to benchmarks by quartiles. Usually, hospitals attempt to stay somewhere between the

TABLE 1.2
Common Financial Terms and Formulas

Term	Abbreviation	Definition	Formula
Adjusted average daily census This number is usually reported for a period of 30 days or greater. As a result, the term used most frequently is adjusted average daily census.	ADJ ADC	The number of inpatients on a unit at midnight and the number of hours outpatients on the unit were in the hospital, divided by 24.	Adjusted patient days plus inpatient census at midnight, divided by the number of days in the selected period. One adjusted patient day = total hours the outpatient surgery patients were in the hospital divided by 24.
Average daily census This number is usually reported for a period of 30 days or greater. As a result, the term used most frequently is average daily census.	ADC	Inpatients in beds at midnight	Total number of inpatients on a unit at midnight for a selected period divided by the number of days in the selected period.
Direct care hours		The number of hours worked by staff in a 24-hour period on a unit This number always includes bedside licensed nurses and aides/technicians. Charge nurses, managers, and/or unit secretaries may be included in some organizations.	Number of caregivers on each shift multiplied by the number of hours in a shift.
Fixed hours		The number of hours worked by staff whose schedules aren't affected by census changes.	The number of people whose schedules don't change according to census multiplied by their assigned hours.
Full-time equivalent	FTE	The number of hours a full-time employee is paid: 2,080 hours a year, 80 hours a pay period, 40 hours a week.	Number of hours worked in a year divided by 2080, or the number of hours worked in a pay period divided by 80.

Term	Abbrev.	Definition	Calculation
Inpatients and outpatients		Patients who are admitted to a bed after midnight and are transferred or discharged before midnight of the admission day.	
Midnight census		The number of inpatients in beds at midnight	The midnight census minus discharges and transfers plus admissions
Nurse–patient ratio		The number of patients assigned to each bedside nurse.	Number of nurses with a care assignment divided by the number of patients at the start of the shift
Paid FTEs	Pd. FTEs	All paid hours divided by the number of hours a full-time person would work in the defined period: 2080 hours a year, 80 hours a pay period, 40 hours a week.	Paid hours in a specified period divided by the number of hours a full-time person would work in that period.
Paid hours	Pd. hrs.	All worked, education, orientation, vacation, holiday, and sick hours in a defined (pay) period.	Add all hours submitted to the payroll system.
Patient days		The length of stay in days	Add the number of midnights each patient stays to determine how many days were accumulated.
Patients per bedside nurse (care nurse)		The number of patients assigned to each bedside nurse. Same as nurse–patient ratio	The number of nurses with a care assignment divided by the number of patients at the start of the shift

(continued)

9

TABLE 1.2 *(continued)*
Common Financial Terms and Formulas

Term	Description	Formula
Productive hours	Any paid hours that are not considered paid time off (vacation, holiday, and sick). Includes worked, education, and orientation hours	Add all hours on the job.
PTO percentage	Number of PTO hours divided by total hours paid.	Number of PTO hours divided by total hours paid.
Target WHPPD	The expected number of hours involved in delivering care to a specific number of patients, including fixed hours.	Select a census number to determine the ideal staffing to care for that patient population in a 24-hour period. Add the fixed staff and divide the census by the new total.
Worked FTEs	Productive or worked hours paid in a period divided by the number of hours a full-time employee would work in the same period.	Add all the hours worked and divide by the number of hours a full-time employee would work.
Worked hours per patient day WHPPD	Worked or productive hours divided by the census in equivalent periods	Add all the hours worked divided by patient days.
Worked hours	Any paid hours that are not considered paid time off (vacation, holiday, and sick). Includes worked, education, and orientation hours. Same as productive hours.	Add all hours on the job.

Note: PTO, paid time off.

50th and 75th quartile. The higher the quartile, the better your productivity is. For example, in a medical floor department in a community hospital, the 50th quartile benchmark may be 18.6 worked hours per equivalent patient day. At the 75th quartile, the benchmark may be 20.72 worked hours per equivalent patient day. Remember that this is measuring the amount of time the staff is delivering care for patients over a 24-hour period. The target for this scenario may be set at about 19.73 worked hours per equivalent patient day if your facility desires to be higher than the 50th quartiles. I have seen hospitals working to improve their quartiles from the 25th or requiring department managers to improve to the 40th or 50th quartile. Monitor your worked hours because they relate to your targets and adjust staffing hours and schedules to stay within budget. Even in busy weeks, take the time to run the numbers and track productivity.

Another area to review daily and weekly is your overtime hours. Many Nurse Managers require prior approval from the manager or supervisor before a staff member can stay beyond their regular work hours. The benchmark for nursing units with overtime is less than 2% of total productive hours. If you find you are trending higher than this level, then look at your staff schedules or review shift change procedures (because this is often where overtime in bedded units occur).

In the next chapter, we offer a simple tool you can use each day to determine the staffing levels you need based on census. The tool also helps calculate your productivity. Whether you use a similar tool or develop your own, managing staffing plans is a major responsibility in your role as a manager.

2

Staffing Models: Managing Capacity to Demand

Nancy Bateman

Trying to determine how many staff is necessary to meet the needs of patients in today's health care system is difficult to do without considering the various staffing models available. No one can predict how many cases or the various levels of acuity that will fall within his or her responsibility on a given day. By using staffing models, Nurse Managers can consider trends and previous statistics to determine future needs without harming budget or acuity. Understanding these models and using them when creating daily staffing plans will ensure that you are managing capacity to meet demand while providing the best quality of care without unnecessary spending.

LEARNING OBJECTIVES

1. Become familiar with different staffing models.
2. Recognize how acuity impacts staffing levels.
3. Be able to achieve flex staffing to demand.

STAFFING TOOLS

There are a variety of tools on the market as well as many home-grown solutions to help manage daily staffing assignments. One of the tools available is an acuity rating system, which provides checklists of required actions per patient. Acuity rating systems can help management determine daily staffing assignments and provide real-time staff availability and patient assignments. Acuity rating systems assume that patients with greater needs will require greater staffing levels because there will be more care-oriented tasks attributed to their well-being. There is some controversy regarding the effectiveness of these systems among Nurse Managers because these systems can be time consuming, can create additional paperwork, and do not always yield results managers expect. Many managers advocate for acuity rating systems when they need additional staff because of more acute patients. However, results of acuity rating systems do not always provide evidence of need.

Other staffing tools are less time consuming to update than acuity rating systems but provide less-precise methods for calculating required staff levels. The staffing template (Table 2.1), which is formulated so that department managers or supervisors only need to enter a daily census, is an initial step in determining which staffing model is best. In this template, benefits (shown always as a percentage of total compensation, obtainable from human resource [HR] or finance departments) are 18%. This template uses California ratios to define the number of professional staff (registered nurses [RNs] or licensed practical nurses [LPNs]) for each shift. Ancillary staff were added using a traditional model of care. The template also calculates the hours per patient day (HPPD) so managers may track their productivity against monthly finance reports. This simple tool is effective when used each afternoon to determine the following day's staffing needs. As we know, most hospitals run a census report at midnight, which does not allow enough time for managers or house nursing supervisors to adjust staffing. By running this model midafternoon daily, staffing adjustments can be performed over the 3:00 p.m. to 11:00 p.m. shift.

The example in Table 2.1 illustrates a 16-bed medical unit, wherein the average daily census (ADC) is 9.6, and staffing accounts for adding an 18% replacement (the number of staff that is out because of vacation or sick time). The model shows a 24/7 factor indicating that this is a weekly staffing plan, and the total full-time equivalents (FTEs) reflect how many staff are needed for the week. This method calculates

TABLE 2.1
Daily Staffing Plan

		RN	LPN	NA	HUC	Total
Number of beds	16					
ADC	9.6					
% Occupancy	60.0					
Projected replacement		18%	18%	18%	18%	
Staff mix		RN	LPN	NA	HUC	Total
Staffing Plan for ADC						
HPPD		5.00	2.50	1.25	0.42	**9.17**
Day		2.00	1.00	0.50	0.50	**4.00**
Evening		2.00	1.00	0.50		**3.50**
Night		2.00	1.00	0.50		**3.50**
24/7 factor		2.40	1.20	0.60	0.20	**4.40**
Replacement		1.51	0.76	0.38	0.13	**2.77**
Total FTEs		**9.91**	**4.96**	**2.48**	**0.83**	**18.17**
Calculated Staffing Plan Ratios						
Day		4.80	9.60	19.20	19.20	
Evening		4.80	9.60	19.20	—	
Night		4.80	9.60	19.20	—	
Average		4.80	9.60	19.20	6.40	

Note: ADC, average daily census; FTE, full-time equivalent; HPPD, hours per patient day; HUC, hospital unit clerk; LPN, licensed practical nurse; NA, nursing assistant; RN, registered nurse.

the staff-ratio plan to prepare for. There is an average of 4.8 patients for each RN, 9.6 patients for each LPN, 19.2 patients per nursing assistant (NA), and one hospital unit clerk (HUC) scheduled only on the day shift. This creates a total weekly staff plan of 18.17 FTEs.

It is important to use one's knowledge of his or her staffing model to develop staffing plans and staff schedules. As daily census figures change, managers will want to adjust staffing levels to maintain agreed-upon ratios.

Staffing Models

A *staffing model* is the structure by which a manager plans a staff schedule. Staffing models determine the ratio of professional nurses to patients required per shift. Support staff includes clinical nurse aides, department or unit secretaries, and materials management support staff for departments such as the emergency department or surgical services. Staffing models also define the roles and tasks of each position as well as staff interactions. The following is a review of available models along with their histories, advantages, and disadvantages.

Primary Care Nursing Model—The *primary care nursing model* is defined as a one-to-one model with a nurse assigned to a patient for the duration of his or her stay. The pros of this model are continuity of care and nurse autonomy during patient care. The primary nurse assumes total responsibility for his or her patient and has the authority to evaluate and coordinate the patient's plan of care with the patient and his or her family members. Use of this model does not mean that each patient must be cared for by an RN; additional nurses or nonlicensed support staff can deliver care under the direction of the patient's primary nurse.

This model is successful with both patients and staff because it allows patients to develop a relationship with their nurse. During the model's introduction in the 1970s and 1980s, patient stays were longer, prompting the need for one-on-one assignments. Additionally, this model thrived as patient symptoms became more complex and included more complicated comorbidities (one or more conditions affecting the health of a patient, which may or may not be related to his or her current diagnosis). Comorbidities were monitored and treated during hospitalization, which supported the need for all-inclusive care plans. For these reasons, primary nurses must be accountable for care plans and must have a broader base of experience, with the ability to reach out to other resources as needed when issues beyond their experience arise.

Continuity of care within this model improves outcomes because communication remains within a smaller network of providers. One primary caregiver is better equipped to define and solve problems because they are recognized earlier. Studies looking at the extent of quality improvements demonstrate differing results—some show improved outcomes, while others found no quantifiable increase in quality or patient well-being (Tiedeman & Lookinland, 2004, pp. 295–296).

In general, the primary care nursing model is more expensive than team nursing. Several professional nurses must be hired to maintain ratios and provide as much bedside care as possible. As with any health care interaction, a patient's perception may rest on the personalities of and the exchanges held with staff. These interactions understandably retain a higher priority when surveyed.

Total Patient Care Model—The total patient care model dates back to the advent of modern nursing and was in use until the early 20th century. This model differs from the primary care nursing model because professional nurses are responsible for administering complete care of their assigned patients throughout the duration of their shift. As shifts change, so do the responsibilities of care to the next charge nurse and nurse provider of care. The charge nurse assigns patients at the beginning of his or her shift, and the assigned nurse provides total care for his or her assignee. The model is more task-centered than decision-driven, as charge nurses are responsible for care coordination, communication, and the recording of patient interactions.

The advantage of this model is higher quality care because it is provided solely by an RN. Because a nurse is assigned to a specific patient, the nurse is able to focus on his or her specific charge with limited distraction. The disadvantage of the model, however, is that care is provided by a single nurse and is therefore only as reliable as the skills and abilities of that designated nurse. Costs for this model are high, and low-priority tasks are performed by highly paid professional nurses. Supporters of the model argue that RNs providing low-priority care can allow for faster diagnoses of newly introduced ailments—concerns that may not be noticed as quickly by non-nurses. Critics would assert, however, that support staff can be trained to recognize these issues and that RNs would pick up on issues during their daily rounds. Studies of this model show conflicting patient and staff satisfaction outcomes. Nurses often cite frustration when caring for a single patient because performing tasks that other less-trained staff could perform prevent them from making the most use of their skill sets. Other nurses, however, enjoy taking care of a single patient at a time, although continuity of care is lost at the end of each shift.

Functional Care Model—Occasionally referred to as *assembly line nursing*; this model is fully task oriented and care is assigned based on skill level. The model is only team oriented from the standpoint of professional and nonprofessional staff working together across all patients. One nurse may be assigned to dispense medications, while nonprofessional support staff may be assigned to less-acute tasks.

From a budgetary standpoint, the functional care model provides a greater use of finances as varying levels of staff are used. With the advent of nursing ratios, this model is not compliant with mandated ratios because lower acuity departments may have high ratios due to the majority of care being provided by nonprofessional staff. Where nursing ratios are not mandated or where there are fewer professional nurses available, this model provides care with the fewest number of RNs.

While some hospitals retained this model during the late 1950s through the early 1970s, its popularity has diminished because of its inherent fragmentation of care. Although cost effective, patients may be delayed in advancing to discharge within this model, eroding any cost savings. Studies show that the model has not provided satisfactory care from neither a patient nor staff perspective. Patients do not build bonds with workers, and professional staff become bored because of task repetition. Nurses do not have a desired level of patient involvement and may feel unable to use their skills properly. From an outcome perspective, this model has the greatest risk of errors and missed opportunities to deliver quality care.

Team Nursing Model—The concept of skilled multilevel teams in patient care emerged in the 1950s. Intending to share responsibility and accountability for patients within a collaborative setting, teams are led by a professional nurse and may be composed of all nurses, or a combination of professional nurses and support staff. In combined teams, an RN provides supervision, evaluation, and addresses levels of care. Team leaders provide very little direct bedside care, however, as teams provide patient care during their shifts.

The team nursing model differs from the primary care nursing model, where responsibilities extend throughout a patient's entire hospital stay. Communication and direction regarding patient care are disseminated from charge nurses to team leaders, and then finally to team members. The effectiveness of the team rests with the leadership and communication style of the team leader. If the team leader supports open communication and sharing of duties, outcomes are decentralized and care outcomes improve. If a team leader is prone to delegate task assignments and communication is limited to team leaders and the charge nurses, then the model resembles the functional care model and suffers from fragmented care.

The cost of implementing the team nursing model is high because of increased staff sizes, and the model is inefficient because of the amount of time spent coordinating care and delegating assignments. The model, however, offers greater continuity of care than the functional care model because it uses varying levels of skilled providers. As a result, patients and staff have more frequent interactions and less staff variation. Team leaders can focus on patient needs, delegating tasks based on the abilities of their team members. It is imperative that team members remain consistent, receiving assignments to the same patients throughout their course of care. Patient and staff perceptions are usually favorable when entire teams work together in this model, fostering patient relationships. Although quality outcomes improve within the functional care model, they are dependent on the team leader's ability to manage staff, communicate with coworkers, and delegate tasks.

Contemporary Nursing Models

Because health care costs rise and nursing ratios are adopted by many hospitals, traditional staffing models have been revised and restructured to accommodate growing patient populations, which require higher levels of care. Hospital administrators have responded to studies proving that employing a greater number of RNs can equate to better outcomes with fewer adverse effects in patient care. Developing balanced approaches to cost and quality concerns have led to the restructuring of traditional care models. Several long-standing concepts use a combination of professional RNs with unlicensed assistant personnel (UAPs), nurse extenders, patient care technicians (PCTs), or certified nurse assistants. These positions are designed to work alongside RNs and provide a comprehensive patient care with a track record of quality outcomes (Tiedeman & Lookinland, 2004). In newer nontraditional models, support staff are trained to supply more than basic patient care; advanced tasks, such as dressing changes, are performed under the direct supervision of RNs. Described in the *Journal of Nursing Administration* as partnered, nonpartnered, nonclinical, and integrated models, the following pairings began appearing in hospitals during the late 1980s because of RN shortages and rising labor costs.

Partnership Clinical Model—The *partnership clinical model* is similar to the team approach, but in this model an RN is partnered with one UAP. As a result of this pairing, the partnership clinical model is also referred to as a *nurse extender model*. Teams are supervised by an RN, with patient groups receiving care from both parties. The UAP is cross-trained to deliver more advanced care than a nurse's aide and functions as a secondary provider of care after the lead RN. The addition of the nonlicensed care provider frees up time for professional nurses to address patient education and assessment. In studies of the model's effectiveness, results were tied to the varying skill and training levels of the unlicensed partner member of the team. Studies on reduced costs from this model showed mixed results because findings did not consider training costs for unlicensed staff. Additionally, most studies showed neither a positive nor a negative impact on patient satisfaction. What's more, most studies were based on RN interviews rather than measurable changes to the baseline of care.

Nonpartnered Clinical Model—Similar to the traditional functional care model, this scenario uses nonlicensed providers performing patient care and other tasks as delegated by RNs without specific, nonchanging pairs. Unlicensed staff may include nursing students, medical students, UAPs, or LPNs. The support staff performs a number of tasks including, but not limited to, taking vitals, patient intake and output, and daily nursing activities.

Nonclinical Model—In this model, UAPs do not perform clinical tasks. Instead, they are responsible for answering calls, delivering water and food trays, and performing all nonclinical work. The addition of a department "hostess" or patient concierge is an effective way to offer patients greater attention and is common within this model. Incorporating a patient concierge into an operating budget can be difficult, however, and many are classified as unit clerks who are also responsible for ordering supplies, transporting equipment, and moving patients.

Integrated Model—As its name suggests, the integrated model uses UAPs for patient care tasks as well as supportive, nonclinical tasks. This model is also referred to as the *professionally advanced care team* (ProACT), a *nurse extender model*, or the *patient care 2000 model* (both of which are expanded within this chapter). The ProACT model was developed at the Robert Wood Johnson Hospital in the 1980s while the hospital experienced widespread nursing shortages and it incorporates elements of the primary care nursing model with RNs acting as care coordinators, and LPNs working alongside UAPs and nurse's aides to provide patient care. Within the integrated model, LPNs fulfill nursing duties when the designated RN is not on duty. Care plans, however, are maintained and established by the RN at all times. As a team manager, RNs are responsible for discharge planning, workload delegation, and care coordination. Although quality improvements have not been studied with this model, most implementations are possible with a neutral impact on operating budgets.

Patient Service Partner Model—The *patient service partner model* is another hybrid model that uses UAPs to support clinical staff while also performing housekeeping, dietary, and food service roles. As in the other nurse extender models, implementation allows RNs to focus on professional care tasks without negatively impacting the quality of care. Studies have shown that patients and staff satisfaction scores are stable within the patient service partner model. In some cases, scores have improved because of the additional personnel made available to share workloads.

Patient Care 2000 Model—Within the *patient care 2000 model*, nurses are supported by PCTs. Unit support specialists fulfill a role similar to that of the nonclinical model, whereas unit support staffs are responsible for housekeeping, ordering supplies, dietary aide duties, and patient transport. The focus of the patient care 2000 model relies on the delegation of duties rather than patient care tasks. The model asserts that more efficient patient care is achieved by reducing staff fragmentation and as a result, many tasks usually provided by outside technicians (electrocardiograms [EKGs], respiratory tests, and physical therapy sessions) are executed by team members within the PCT. Given that PCTs also function as nurse extenders, full-time employee expenses for hospital units are also reduced. Currently, outcomes from this model have not been studied with adequate sample sizes (Lookingland, Tiedeman, & Crosson, 2005).

Before discussing the *flex staffing model*, it is important to review another important role within traditional and nontraditional models. As the highlighted models are structurally similar, the role of a clinical care manager proves critical to reducing the lengths of patient stays, errors in care, and improved patient satisfaction. Although case management is a long-standing element of patient care, previous iterations were similar to roles executed by utilization nurses until the current revision of models began. True case management models provide clinical coordination between nursing, medical, social work, and ancillary services. Case management models should be either unit-based, with managers assigned to specific floors, or disease-based, with managers assigned to specific disease categories. The most important aspects of patient care within these models are reductions in staff variability and improved communication. Case managers can bridge communication and care gaps, ensuring that patient care is consistent across all interactions through coordinated efforts.

Case management programs should include a department manager who is responsible for implementation and daily operation. A manager, often an RN or social worker, works collaboratively with key physicians to ensure attainment of goals, as well as compliance to policies and procedures, communicating results to both physicians and hospital administrators. Additionally, managers are responsible for screening admissions, managing resources, planning discharges, and facilitating hand-offs. Case managers play a vital role in the delivery of total patient care because they are charged with coordinating care across the continuum. In most programs, case managers should have a ratio of 1:25–30 patients. While reporting results and communicating care efforts, case managers also serve as key liaisons between physicians, nurses, and interdisciplinary teams.

Social workers are also important to the success of a team operating within the case management model, because they support patients through multiple levels of inpatient and nonacute care. Social workers can initiate referrals to protective services in cases of suspected abuse or neglect, serve as consultants in power-of-attorney scenarios, facilitate adoption plans, and can advance directives for patients. Responsible for psychosocial intervention, crisis intervention, and the mobilization of community services, social workers should have a ratio of 1:40–60 patients and ensure access to appropriate community and financial resources when patients are discharged.

> **Flex Staffing Model**—The common nursing term *capacity to demand* refers to the need for flexibility on a shift-to-shift basis, meeting patient demands, and maintaining the capacity to provide effective care. Anyone admitted to an emergency department for care can understand the need for space (capacity) to meet the needs (demand) of patients. The nature of health care, however, is destined to be inconsistent: If one could know that each Thursday night would host five patients with chest pain, two teens with broken bones, and six children with chest colds, health care providers would be prepared and staffed with an appropriate number of nurses, doctors, and support staff that have the skills required to treat the population. Because forecasting with this level of specificity is not possible, it is imperative to equip floors with as many professional and support staff members as possible, training for as many different types of patient complaints as is practical.

It is possible to track census measurements of available staff and beds within a floor, which can help identify peak usage hours and account for spikes in patient admissions. Emergency, respiratory, radiology, and surgical services departments all see patients as they flow through a hospital. As such, these departments are referred to as *nonbedded units* because patients are usually on gurneys and not assigned to particular beds until assigned to hospital rooms. Patient floors, where room and bed assignments are made for each admitted patient, are therefore referred to as *bedded units*. Bedded units are easier to predict for staffing because of the finite number of rooms and beds available. Once a bedded department is full, patients assigned to that department are held at their current department until a patient is discharged or transferred, thus freeing a bed for a new patient.

Census tracking within bedded units can provide an excellent indicator of staff capacity. If a department has 10 patient rooms with two beds apiece, then the department's capacity is 20 patients. By maintaining accurate ADC figures, caregivers can keep track of the comings and goings of admitted patients. Because patients are sent home as soon as possible, staffing schedules are based on average census figures. If a department is at 90% census, 18 patients are currently within the department's oversight and care. Conversely, if a report states that the census is at 110%, this indicates that there are admitted patients who are awaiting the transfer or discharge of others before being placed in a room. In this scenario, patients may wait in hallways on gurneys while beds are cleaned or made available. Additionally, this census can indicate that a department has extra rooms that are not usually staffed—and because of a temporary crisis or volume expansion—put beds back into use. When taking census figures, it is important to note the difference between "licensed" beds and "staffed" beds. Many hospitals are licensed for more beds than they schedule staff to cover and, as a result, department directors may opt to close a number of beds if there is no anticipated need to staff them. While these beds are still licensed, they are not staffed and should not be included within census figures.

Another important consideration when choosing between staffing models is patient acuity. Most patients admitted today are higher in acuity than ever before. Because many complaints and issues can be treated through an urgent or outpatient care, admitted patients are usually in greater need of care. An acuity tool is helpful in identifying and tracking patient progression as well as the department manager's or supervisor's need to assign an adequate level of nursing skill to each patient. There are several acuity tools available for purchase, usually tying into the day-to-day activities of departmental staff members. Table 2.2 is a sample of this type of tool.

Armed with a basic understanding of different models, many administrators seek out other hybrid models that are part of ongoing research. New research models emerge as administrators seek cost savings without negative impacts on safety and patient outcomes. Staffing ratios and census figures play a large part in the development of burgeoning models, owing to the budgetary concerns faced by many hospitals. A recent study on the outcomes of quality and nurse satisfaction compared nursing ratios in California, Pennsylvania, and New Jersey, finding that "hospital nurse staffing ratios mandated in California are associated with lower mortality and nurse outcomes predictive of better nurse retention in California and in other states where they occur" (Aiken et al., 2010, p. 1). Research for this article was conducted as a survey that used data from 22,336 hospital staff nurses and discharge databases in California, Pennsylvania, and New Jersey, all of which were obtained in 2006. Results of the survey noted that implementation of California's ratios resulted in nurses caring for one less patient than within the other surveyed states. The study noted a decrease in mortality and improved quality outcomes, with lowered instances of nurse burnout and job dissatisfaction (Aiken et al., 2010).

When the Patient Protection and Affordability Care Act (PPACA) comes into effect in October 2012, Centers for Medicare and Medicaid Services (CMS) reimbursements may change in many hospitals, affecting the ability of health care providers to meet quality measure scores on 17 clinical processes of care and eight dimensions of the patient care experience. Although the mandates of PPACA may change and other elements may be added, it is clear that quality outcomes and safety are going to remain a priority and will be tied to reimbursements upon the introduction of the Act's legislation. As a result, budgeting is a crucial consideration when adapting a nursing model. A unit's budget should be based on several assumptions. Although some staffing numbers are fixed, such as the number of Nurse Managers and unit clerks, others are flexible and should be based on workloads. For example, if there is only one room open on a floor, there will be a smaller number of staff on duty than if there were five rooms open. In either case, there will still only be one manager and one unit clerk on duty. In addition to the impact of patient volume on staffing numbers, patient acuity is also an important factor. If there are 10 patients in an inpatient medical unit and patients are also in an ICU, more staff will be needed in the ICU where patient acuity is higher and direct care is more necessary. Because of these budgetary considerations, Nurse Managers and nurse directors work with finance departments to establish an appropriate number of FTEs, budgeted salary workers, and budgeted productivity metrics (such as worked care HPPD).

With this information in mind, it is important to investigate the flex staffing model as introduced earlier in the chapter. When departments are able to flex their

TABLE 2.2
Patient Classification System—Medical Surgical, Progressive Care, Mother Baby Units

	Level 1	Level 2	Level 3	Level 4	Level 5
Vital signs	Unit routine Weigh, one person to assist Pulse oximetry		Q2 hours Weigh, two people to assist		Hourly Weigh, three or more people to assist
ADL—bath	Minimal assistance		Partial assistance		Total bath
ADL—toilet	Self-toileting		Assist to toilet or Foley		Incontinent
ADL—feeding			Assistance		
Activity	Walk with assistance BID, up in chair		Turn and position Q2 hours		Up in chair or walking with two or more people to assist
Orientation			Disoriented		Wandering and pulling tubes, no sitter Demanding mental health issues
Language			Language/speech barrier without intervention		Language/speech barrier with intervention
Medication	IVPB and PO meds Routine BSG, insulin sliding scale		Multiple IVPB, IV push Repeated BSG, more than routine		Titrated drips BSG hourly
			IV chemo administration		Intraperitoneal chemo or first dose chemo
	PO or PCA pain control				Uncontrolled pain
IV	One line or lock		Double/triple lumen, central line, chemo port		
Procedures			Blood administration		
	Continuous central monitoring		Continuous monitoring		Arrhythmias triggering alarm
	Durable medical equipment		Initial set up, durable medical equipment		

TABLE 2.2 *(continued)*

	Level 1	Level 2	Level 3	Level 4	Level 5
Procedures			G to J tube for feeding or meds Invasive procedure this shift Chest tube		
				Restraints or high risk for fall	
			Palliative care, grief issues		
			Ostomy, wound care, dressing drains		
	Oxygen		CPAP, BiPAP		
			Trach care/ suctioning		
				Isolation	
Teaching	Prepared program or materials		New diagnosis, education support		
			Teaching with return demonstration		
	2 points each		**4 points each**		**5 points each**

Note: ADL, activities of daily living; BID, twice a day; BiPAP, bilevel positive airway pressure; BSG, blood sugar glucose; CPAP, continuous positive airway pressure; G tube, gastrostomy; IV, intravenous; IVPB, intravenous piggyback; J tube, jejunostomy; PCA, patient-controlled analgesia; PO, by mouth; Q2 hours, every 2 hours.

staffing based on daily census counts, they are free to meet demand capacity with appropriately trained staff members. Although health care providers with specific skills may be needed during a portion of an average workday, they will be free for use elsewhere when not in high demand. This model allows floors to use specialists without creating staffing redundancies—allowing employees with specific skill sets to work in various settings as needed.

APPLYING THE FLEX STAFFING MODEL TO LABOR AND PRODUCTIVITY

Structuring an approach should be a key focus when deciding on a staffing model. The chosen approach must offer a real-time productivity monitoring system for labor and nonlabor expenses that is also sensitive to fluctuations in volume. The flex staffing model offers both real-time productivity monitoring as well as cost savings for ongoing labor resources, reducing the use of temporary, traveling, and agency staff. A successfully implemented flex staffing model offers tools that

■ provide flexible volume forecasting and budgeting processes,
■ design variable staffing plans,
■ develop criteria for use of agency/supplemental staff,
■ link budgeting, staffing, and scheduling,
■ identify and quantify approaches for factors affecting productivity (e.g., acuity, skill/competency levels, workload fluctuations), and
■ provide effective and easy to use tools for ongoing measurement.

The clinical flex staffing model builds upon the traditional flex staffing model, including a productivity model that divides performance measures by bedded and nonbedded units. Nonbedded units include surgical and emergency departments, radiology, catheterization labs, and interventional radiology units. A particularly successful approach can be found within a flexible staffing model that incorporates an expanded float pool. In this framework, roles and responsibilities for several key positions are revised to include staffing coordinators, bed placement, and float pool departments. These areas have been shown to provide significant impact within a short time frame and minimal effort. To pursue this approach, it is important to determine a monthly baseline for admissions and discharges, reviewing existing staffing plans compared to daily census measurements. This assessment identifies trends in utilization and management strategies, measuring fluctuations in service units and length-of-stay reductions. The approach incorporates the following:

■ **Forecasting demand:** Establish expected departmental utilization (patient days) based on key planning assumptions (growth) and anticipated changes in volume (changes on lengths of stay).
■ **Trending volume:** Identify volume changes by years, months, and days. Identify significant changes and influencing factors (seasonal, physician practices, program changes, etc.).
■ **Managing resources:** Review trends regularly to improve predictability of utilization/demand. Identify potential changes in volume before they happen.

In addition to monitoring the daily census, it is important to also track patient acuity and patient flow. When reviewing staffing needs, it is important to include admissions, discharges, and other elements crucial to patient flow within a unit. Figure 2.1 provides an example of how to track admissions and discharges, thereby developing a staffing plan with a float pool. The figure accommodates high levels of admission and discharge overlap throughout the day.

The flex staffing model not only focuses on tasks in a manner similar to traditional team approaches, but also allocates staff for the duration of a patient's hospital stay because staff can be flexed to fit census needs based on daily figures. Although staff members should be informed of their schedules according to existing policies, core staffing is still reduced to maintain pace with daily census figures over the

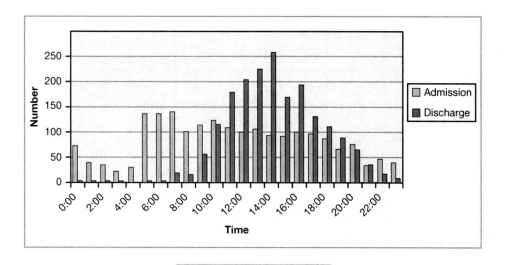

FIGURE 2.1
Admissions and Discharges for October 2001

course of a full year because these figures are not related to the number of staffed beds. Core staff numbers should be tied to the lowest average census figure, not including nurses required for special treatments, orientation, training, or backfilling for paid time off, or daily work breaks. These job functions are handled through the use of the expanded float pool.

A key component to successful adaption of this model is the coordination of the staffing coordinator, bed manager, unit-based clinical care manager, and department manager.

Use of the flex staffing model tracks productivity by position, shift, and daily census. An advantage of the flex staffing model besides the expanded float pool is the ability to track compliance and accountability. Current productivity tools can be manipulated to report higher productivity based on acuity assignments and use of staff for orientation and training. The flex staffing model uses float pool staff for these tasks, and acuity is an integral part of the staffing ratios so adherence to the ratios fulfills the acuity assignments. This becomes a nonissue with regard to accuracy of level assignments.

In developing a flex staffing model, the float pool is expanded with levels of care delivery. Special divisions are created for medical and surgical floors, intensive care unit (ICU), and telemetry and surgical services, aligning support staff within the created divisions. The staffing tool uses daily census to determine staffing ratios and also calculates actual HPPD on a real-time basis. Staffing is adjusted daily based on bed occupancy, and flex staffing for the next day is decided before the end of the day shift each day. The expanded float pool services the divisions they support, allowing for a greatly reduced base level or "core" staffing.

Most hospitals run a census report at midnight. This is fine for finance reporting but to staff a department effectively based on daily census and acuity, the next day's staffing should be evaluated by 3:00 p.m. on the current day. With a core staffing level that is based on staffed beds, staffing levels do not need to be as lean as the flex staffing model. When there is a light census day, core staff can do other tasks. This does not mean that staff from the float pool cannot be pulled to free up core staffing and complete other administrative tasks. What it does mean is that the patient population is cared for with less use of temporary and agency staff and also allows for times when staffing levels are lower. The flex staffing model also helps with overtime because float pool staff can be pulled for as little as one hour or as long as a full 12-hour shift.

Many factors affect the ability of a department to use flex resources effectively. If the department has a variable skill mix, the ability to flex is higher. Patient care can be assigned to higher skilled staff; Nurse Managers can and do backfill with float staff. A variable skill mix also allows managers to match caregiver skills to patient/population requirements. The percentage of part-time staff affects how one would use a flex staffing model because higher percentages of part-time staff provide a greater ability to respond to rapid fluctuations in census (60:40). While most managers would agree, they prefer full-time versus part-time staff, or per-diem staff; this does allow greater flexibility, and adaption of the flex staffing model is easier.

For departments with specialized skills such as the cardiac catheterization lab, emergency departments, or surgical services, the flex staffing model has department and skill specific float pools. The percentage of on-call requirements affects how the flex staffing model is implemented but does not affect the success of the model.

To adapt the model, current policies and procedures, which may impact the flexibility or impose restrictions in moving resources between units, needs to be reviewed. Even in facilities that are highly unionized, the model has been adapted and remains successful years later.

The Staffing Coordinator Role Shift

The greatest change with the flex staffing model is the role of the staffing coordinator. Most existing staffing coordinators are responsible for inputting staff schedules in an electronic database, verifying staff coming in, reconciling schedules to incoming staff, and finding staff to backfill the incoming shifts. Routinely, they communicate with the charge nurses for an early census between 9:00 and 11:00 a.m., and then again in the afternoon for the next three shifts. Usually they verify census and staffing needs by 1:00 p.m., and by 2:00 p.m., an assessment is made to see how to staff shifts, and for a low census, what staff to call off.

The future role of a staffing coordinator is much more involved and often will require a review of the current job description to accommodate the added responsibilities. In the future role, the responsibilities are expanded to function as an RN coach who works with unit managers and assistant unit managers. The coaching role is to educate management on scheduling of staff, with daily staffing assignments for the right skill set according to patient needs and acuity. The future role must be the liaison between administration and department managers for the bigger view by person, department, and hospital wide as it relates to census and staffing needs. The staffing coordinator is also the supervisor for the float pool. This position now covers a highly expanded float pool with its layers of skill and specialties.

Current float pools often have as few as three RNs and possibly one to two nurse aides or UAPs. Float pools routinely do not have unit secretaries or clerks as part of the mix. With a flex staffing model, the float pool includes a predetermined number of RNs, LPNs, and operating room (OR), cardiac, and critical care–certified professional staff, as well as one to two unit clerks managed by a staffing coordinator and one to two staffing clerks.

The staffing coordinator is a critical position for expanded float pools to work especially when implementing a flex staffing model. The staffing coordinator is responsible for assigning the appropriate level of staff to each request, tracking the assignments so as much consistency as possible is provided daily to the same inpatients, and making rounds on the floors twice a day to personally assess the needs in number of staff, staff skills, and duration of assignment. The advantage of a flex staffing model is that a floor does not require to be position filled for the entire 8- or 12-hour shift if added help is only required during lunch relief or to perform special procedures.

The difference between a staffing coordinator's duties today compared to what the new responsibilities will transition to are outlined as follows:

Current Role

- Input schedules into the electronic database
- Verify and reconcile incoming staff schedules
- Find staff for the next shift
- Talk to charge nurses for an early census between 9:00 and 11:00 a.m., and then again in the afternoon for the next three shifts
- Verify census and staffing needs at 1:00 p.m. daily
- Assess staff shifts and census figures at 2:00 p.m. daily

Future Role

- RN coach who works with unit managers and support staff
- Scheduling coaching
- Daily staffing assignment coaching
- Greater role for the manager and support staff to staff the unit on a real-time basis—routine look ahead
- Assume a wide-ranging assessment of staffing needs
- Revised management of float pool

When considering personality types for the role, begin by seeking a staffing coordinator with a proactive and assertive attitude, high-energy approach, and a willingness to make important decisions. The success of the expanded flex staffing model requires the strength of the staffing coordinator and the structure—whether through information management or a simple but effective spreadsheet that can be updated for every shift—so that staffing needs are met with the right skills and the required timing.

Let's look at what a typical day in the life of a staffing coordinator would be like.

A Day in the Life of a Flex Model Staffing Coordinator

- Works a 9:00 a.m.-to-5:00 p.m. shift
- Reports directly to chief nursing officer (CNO)

- Oversees staffing office, bed manager, and admissions team
- Staffing is flexed to census with staffing requirements determined by 4:00 p.m. daily (In absence of staffing coordinator, house supervisor is in charge.)
- The position is one of importance with unit managers working closely with the staffing coordinator
- Staffing coordinator or staffing clerk makes rounds twice per day
- Expanded float pool is managed by staffing department
- Next day assignments are communicated by 6:00 p.m. the night before for per diem staff

The Role of Float Pools in the Flex Staffing Model

The following is an example of a float-pool offering to current full-time employees:

Float-Pool Employment Option
- Current float-pool employees with guaranteed hours will have two employment options evaluated quarterly
- Current employment options:
  1. Maintain current job status (full time, part time, per diem) without any changes
  2. Move to the new float pool as outlined in the following text or unit-based per diem model under discussion
  3. New hires or anyone changing current job status to float pool will move to the new float pool

The New Float Pool
- PRN, no guarantee of hours
- Float to many units (based on qualifications)
- Required to declare availability for a minimum of 36 to 40 hours a month, 60 days ahead of the first day of the next schedule:
  - 12 to 16 hours of availability must be Saturday or Sunday
- Required to declare availability for two holidays:
  - Thanksgiving, Christmas, or New Year
  - Memorial Day, Independence Day, or Labor Day
- In times of low census float pool, staff are canceled after overtime staff and before straight time full-time, part-time, and per-diem staff
- May work for a full-time, part-time, or per-diem staff if the shift is in addition to the schedule days and with the prior approval of the Nurse Manager
- Base pay is the midpoint of salary range of the job title plus 30%
- Eligible for all applicable shift differentials
- Not eligible for any benefits

- Each individual in the float pool will be noted at 0.01 FTE within the float-pool cost center.
- The number of people in the float pool will not exceed:
  - 40 RNs
  - 6 LPNs
  - 12 Tech/NAs
  - 2 Support staff
- If a float-pool member works 80 hours in one cost center/department in 6 months, the staffing coordinator completes the evaluation of the float-pool staff members after reviewing performance with the unit manager or assistant unit manager (AUM). This input will be reviewed with the float-pool member and returned to the float pool office for filing. At annual evaluation time, these evaluations will be considered as input into the annual performance review.
- Nonavailability or failure to work in any given 30-day period will result in termination.

The Use of Sitters in the Flex Staffing Model

A small component to managing staff, but one that often can create issues with staffing is the occasional need for a "sitter." A sitter is an employee who must stay with a patient at all times, usually for suicide watch. Hospitals often ask a family member to sit with the patient, but doing so creates an issue of legal responsibility if something were to happen to the patient while being "watched" by the family member. A good sitter policy and use of the float pool can diminish any disruptions of staff levels or care delivery if a structured policy is in place. The following is an example of a sitter policy.

Sitter Policy and Procedure
Purpose
1. Procedural steps to follow when obtaining sitters
2. Uniform performance expectations for employees
3. Uniform performance expectations for others

Writing the Policy and Procedure
- Use flow chart to guide procedure steps
  - Care nurse should contact family member(s) when in-house sitter care is considered
  - Nonemployee sitters are oriented to the hospital and explained expectations by the care nurse
  - RN assessment of nonemployee sitter capabilities must be documented in the patient record
  - Use of a handout for nonemployee sitters should include a signature/date line and RN signature line to confirm the information was given to the sitter

Sitter Protocols/Duties

Hospital employees are to perform all duties associated with their role (RN, LPN, and nursing assistant certified [NAC]) for up to three patients in the same geographic/ visual setting. This includes:

■ activities of daily living (ADL)

■ vital signs

■ toileting

■ walking

■ charting

Others (i.e., family members, sitters from other agencies):

■ call the nurse

■ sign in and out with care nurse

■ stay awake and attentive

■ feed the patient

■ reorient the patient

Other responsibilities that may be done after assessment of the sitter capabilities might include

■ toileting

■ bathing

■ ADL

When matching capacity to demand it is important to have a thorough understanding of the various staffing models. Refer back to the descriptions of these models to create schedules that meet acuity. Understanding the history, advantages, and disadvantages of the available models will ensure that your ability to meet demand is efficient and productive.

SUMMARY

Understanding various staffing models and considering their advantages and disadvantages can help managers make tough decisions when it comes to the quality of care offered within a department. A thorough understanding of staffing models is required to manage staff. Acuity ratings and the ability to extend them into staffing assignments further increases the productivity and quality of a department. Be sure to report all productivity plans and variances to administration so staffing remains in alignment with capacity and demand.

3

Recruitment and Dismissals

Nancy Bateman

Finding the right skill sets and levels of experience to fill vacant positions is as much a challenge as being faced with the need to dismiss an employee. In all cases, you need the guidance of your human resources (HR) representative. Although he or she can guide you in the areas of protocol and policy, it will be up to you as the department manager to evaluate a new hire's fit with your needs.

LEARNING OBJECTIVES

1. Assess skills required when recruiting.
2. Recognize personality as a factor in successful hiring.
3. Employ the process for dismissing an employee.

RECRUITING

Defining Required Staff Skills

When you begin to address filling a position, it is helpful to be involved in the creation or review of the job posting. You should also begin by reviewing the job description for the open position. It is at this time you can make adjustments if needed. Adjustments could be in the form of requiring the ability to flex schedules or you may be looking to fill a night position or 12-hour shift. These should be clearly defined in the job posting.

Depending on the position being filled (i.e., professional nurse or support staff), it is an option to develop a simple sample patient scenario to test for knowledge and/ or computer skills. Combined with the interview, this can flush out the differences in interpretation of skill levels. I remember interviewing a registered nurse (RN) for a consulting position that required a great deal of experience in analytics and Excel spreadsheets. When asked what level of skill she had in analytics, she described herself as very skilled. Once she was on board, we found that she was able to review spreadsheets but had no idea how to work within a spreadsheet. When asked about her previous statement on her skill levels, she remarked that she always had someone else prepare the spreadsheets and do any changes. In her mind, the interview was focused on her clinical knowledge and her ability to interpret the analytics in the spreadsheet versus the need to be able to operate the software. It was a hard lesson learned on both sides, and I have since developed and used sample case studies to test the candidate so we both understand the work involved and the skill level definitions.

For a direct patient care provider, it is also advised to request even seasoned professional staff to demonstrate basic skills. Depending on the length of your orientation and mentoring program, gaining a baseline of performance skills may help when deciding between multiple recruits. This approach also ensures that the resume is of the level expected.

As a department manager or a staff nurse asked to assist with interviews, you should be familiar with not just the skill sets already in place in your unit but also the personalities and culture of the unit. Often it isn't only a priority to fill the position with a similar education and preparation, but also to keep the dynamics of the overall team intact or upgraded.

A component to consider when choosing who should fill the vacancy is a concept found in an article published by the *Harvard Business Review*. I found the article in the *US Airways* flight magazine when I was on a recent business trip. The article was called "What 17th-Century Pirates Can Teach Us About Job Design." It describes the impact when the wrong people are hired for the wrong reasons. The article starts with the importance of building the job description so that people with the right mix of aptitudes will be applying for the job. It is also important to understand how the right applicant will fulfill the specific tasks of the open position. This concept goes back to the culture and personalities of the unit more than the basic knowledge and experience of the interviewee.

In the article, Harvard MBA students were asked to think about the history of pirates and to develop a job description for the captain of a pirate ship. The students came up with skills for the position that were defined as a combination of star tasks and guardian tasks. The *star tasks* involved strategy, negotiation skills, and command during battle. The *guardian tasks* were more aligned with operational duties including distribution of supplies and organizing care for the sick and injured. If you think about the people you currently work with you should see the same comparisons as I did. In your unit or any place of work, you have personalities that can quickly size up an issue and develop a plan of action. The same individuals are more apt to approach a difficult physician and negotiate a plan of care for their patients. They are stronger in leadership skills and they voice their opinions. The guardians are the persons who jump in and get the work done. They are the peacekeepers and go the extra mile for the care of their patients. Star tasks belong to the risk takers and entrepreneurs; guardian tasks are for those who are conscientious and systematic. While both types are admiral and needed, the author of the article believes it is difficult to find people who are equally good in both types. I tend to agree with him (Rao, 2010).

As it relates to filling your vacant position, you would be wise to take these two personality types into consideration with your current mix of staff. Remember the old adage, "Too many cooks?" or "Too many chiefs?" In modern times, the title of star task might go to your CEO, whereas the title of guardian task would go to your COO. In all layers of an organization, you can pick out the CEOs and the COOs. If you think about the people you work with, you can assign these traits to them as well. Filling a support role or an RN's position requires the right mix of skill, knowledge, and experience. But as you interview the candidates, evaluate their personality traits for the dynamics of the team. Hiring a star when you know you have many on the team already could cause conflict. If the candidate is required to excel in both traits, he or she will gravitate to the more comfortable type anyway; so in using the case study test examples, you might consider adding questions or scenarios to the case example that will evaluate the candidate's tendency toward star tasks or guardian tasks. Your unit's culture is like a family unit, and keeping it balanced will support staff satisfaction and retention.

Another option to consider when interviewing for a position within your department is to invite the candidate to join several team members for lunch. This is usually done for higher levels of responsibility; however, it allows initial interactions with the recruit and team members. It doesn't hurt to have several strong staff participate in the assessment of an individual's ability to fill a vacancy on the team.

During your one-on-one interview, a professional yet friendly approach allows the recruit to relax and present his or her best offering. I have interviewed nurses and support staff who were so nervous they could hardly speak, yet they can answer questions with clear and accurate answers. Once they begin to relax, you can continue the interview and gain insight into their problem-solving approach and personality traits. I am more interested in their ability to demonstrate their knowledge, experience, and desire to provide a high degree of patient care than impressing me with overconfidence.

There are many interview guides available on the Internet and probably available from your HR or education department. The usual guide includes scenarios where you ask the recruits how they would handle a difficult situation or to describe a time when they realized they had made a mistake and what they did about it. I think these are good examples to use along with the technical review. Be prepared with several questions directly related to the work they will perform on your unit. If you are interviewing multiple candidates, it does help to ask each recruit the same questions. Although your interview may sway into other areas of discussion, having a common thread to your interview allows you to better rate one recruit over another.

IMPORTANCE OF PERFORMANCE DOCUMENTATION AND REVIEWS

As a busy Nurse Manager, annual performance reviews may seem like a begrudging task. Try looking at this effort as a way to strengthen your entire team while providing career growth for your staff. Most of us have been trained on how to interact with our colleagues. I have always heard that you need to start discussions with positive remarks and then discuss or list areas for improvements. I don't think the order of the documentation and discussions really matters, as we all know we will cover both positives and negatives. You do need to recognize the areas of strength each staff member exhibits and if this strength is consistent. However, you also need to use this time to discuss any area where further education, training, or behavior modification is warranted.

The more difficult review is when behavior is an issue. Personality conflicts can be improved with team building activities and these are discussed in Chapter 11.

When an individual has colleagues complaining about attitude or policies and rules are not complied with, then it is imperative that the conflicts and your discussions be well documented.

I have dealt with individuals whose poor behavior has been ignored. There comes a time when corrective action is needed, and the ability to improve the situation is delayed without the proper documentation. Consider, for example, a staff member who routinely treats his or her colleagues with condescending comments. By the time the situation is elevated to the Nurse Manager, the behavior may have been long term because coworkers have decided to ignore the individual rather than make a complaint. When a staff treats others without respect and professionalism, the working environment is disrupted, which reduces the quality of care delivered. If you are an engaged manager you will notice this behavior. If the situation is reported to you then documentation of the complaint is required. Follow up with the individual and offer to hear his or her side of the story. Some managers like to bring in both parties to sit and discuss the issues. I find this only works when it is a personality conflict between two colleagues. General complaints or multiple complaints require one-on-one follow-up.

If the issue is lack of compliance to policy or rules, then this also needs to be addressed and documented. Written detail of the issues and plans for corrective actions with timelines for improvements provides a paper trail and the ability to return to the discussion to track changes.

All issues discussed and documented require two points. The first is a detailed report of the discussion. Date and time—both at the start of the discussion and the end of the discussion to document the length of time spent with the individual. The second point is to make improvements measurable. In the case of the person who has been disrespectful to his or her coworkers, it may be necessary to survey the staff to report if they see improvement. Requesting the individuals to take it on themselves to approach colleagues and openly offer to discuss the perceived behavior may help. For lack of compliance to policy and rules, the measurable improvements are easier as the individuals can record when they have shown compliance.

For all annual reviews or quarterly reviews, staff are to be held accountable to all provisions of their roles. During preparation for their reviews, staff should prepare a file that demonstrates compliance, any contributions they have made to the team or department, and any new education or training. The manager should prepare his or her own file for each reviewee with time and attendance, compliance to required skills inventories, and participation in department or hospital committees.

Reviews should be scheduled far enough in advance so staff arrives prepared. Clear expectations on what preparations are requested are communicated at the time the review is scheduled. Offering an example of the file you will review allows both sides to prepare an adequate file. Showing them the elements that will be reviewed reduces their apprehension, as they will go into the meeting with a known agenda.

If areas for improvement are documented with measurable corrective actions, then monthly meetings to review progress keep the individual on track.

When performing annual reviews for solid performers use this annual review to help the staff members create a career development plan. If your hospital has a career ladder program there may be specific items listed that were developed to support career advancement. Whether you have set career ladders or not, you can work with the staff within your own department to identify management tasks or areas of advancing responsibilities they can undertake. Many of the tasks you perform weekly can be delegated to a member of your team who desires to learn advancement skills. These may be staff scheduling, calculating weekly productivity, or training for a role as mentor. These tasks should be repeatable, such as the staff scheduling, so the staff becomes proficient and accuracy and knowledge increase. Once you have trained them and routinely check their work, you can add this task to their responsibilities. The process helps lighten your workload of routine responsibilities while supporting career growth for the interested staff.

When creating the career path, make sure you check with your supervisor and have the delegated tasks communicated to him or her. You want the support to assign the responsibilities to the interested staff and ensure that the work they will do for you counts when they are considered for a promotion.

A final suggestion for advancing your staff is to post a list of opportunities for career advancement along with the annual review schedules so more than one staff member can discuss with you different areas that are of interest to him or her. You may have a few who would like to advance in education or mentoring, whereas others would like to take the management path. These areas for advancement should be communicated often and discussed quarterly in team member meetings because you would not want to delay staff interest by waiting for the annual review period.

PERFORMANCE IMPROVEMENT PLANS

When all else fails and improvements are not achieved, or when behaviors or skills present serious issues, then placing the individual on a performance improvement plan (PIP) is the next step. Unless the issue is a cause for immediate dismissal, your employee is usually given the opportunity to participate in a formal and structured plan. Check with your HR department for the approved process. Usually, the term for the PIP is as short as one month or as long as six months. The majority of PIPs that I have used are one to three months. The timeline is related to needs. If an individual needs additional training to remain in his or her role, the length of the PIP should account for the time required to complete the training.

When the issues are behavioral, I prefer a shorter term. Unless the behavior can be corrected or improved quickly, you risk retention of your stronger staff. PIPs are a confidential agreement between you as the manager and the individual, with specific areas for focused change and measurable milestones documenting improvement. While the rest of your team should not be aware of the PIP, they should quickly see visible changes in behavior.

The first step in the process is to speak with your HR representative. He or she can advise you on the hospital policy. I mentioned time frames for the PIP; however, your HR policy may dictate the required length. If the timeline is longer than you are comfortable with, you can discuss this with your chief nursing officer (CNO) or require the individual to schedule monthly update meetings and stay close to the process.

If you have adequate and consistent documentation from prior reviews, the personal file will support the PIP, and communicating the plan to the individual should not be a surprise. If the situation is relatively new and grievous enough to require an immediate PIP, then I would suggest asking your HR representative to be present when you introduce the plan to the individual. If the PIP is related to disruptive behavior it would be good to have HR present as well.

Most PIPs are in the form of a written report with details including dates and times of examples representing the issues. When complaints are involved the HR representative will interview the parties prior to completing the report so all information is included. The staff member who has submitted the complaints should be kept confidential. The individuals being placed on the PIP should be advised that they are prohibited from asking or investigating who may have submitted the complaints, and any attempt at retaliation will be cause for immediate action.

The plan will have specific requirements for improvement and timelines for each step in the process. I have to admit that in my experience most people when placed on improvement plans either quit or fail to improve to the point of completing the plan. I believe this is due to leadership waiting too long to use a PIP. Rather than use a PIP as a last attempt to make needed changes, the better approach is to stay engaged with your staff and use performance reviews as originally intended.

DISMISSAL OF A STAFF MEMBER

Finally, hiring is a difficult process, but dismissing an employee is very stressful. The wisest advice is to follow the protocol from your HR liaison and complete the process as quickly as you can, following the determination that it needs to be done.

Before an individual can be terminated the decision needs to be approved by your supervisor. HR should ensure all protocol has been met. Documentation of the actions taken prior to the decision is critical. If the individual has been on a PIP, written updates will support the lack of progress. Without a PIP the final file should clearly state the reasons for the decision.

You should have the HR representative with you when you meet with the individual. Many times this is completed by your CNO or service line leader, but if the process rests with you it is important to be professional, discreet, and make the meeting short. Dwelling on the decision-making process or creating a situation where the individual cannot finish the meeting and be released in a timely manner is embarrassing for him or her and only heightens a difficult situation. No matter what the reason for the dismissal, the employee deserves respect and enough explanation so he or she is clear on the reason for the dismissal. I suggest rehearsing the discussion with your supervisor and HR so you stay within protocol.

Communicating to your team that an individual is no longer employed should be simple and without detail. If the team was aware of issues they can figure it out for themselves. Your role is not to participate in the gossip that may be present. As a leader your team will respect the fact that you handled the situation professionally.

A final word on dismissing an employee: People handle stress in many ways, and you may try to predict how the individual will react, and you may be wrong. If the dismissal is caused by aggressive behavior you certainly should have HR present and may even ask security to stand by to escort the individual off the premises. You may not know what is happening in this person's personal life, so even mild-mannered people can react "out of character" when confronted with losing their employment. Always alert HR and security when you are scheduling a meeting to dismiss an employee. Allow the individual time to clean out his or her locker or desk but also instruct him or her to complete the task within the hour and leave the premises. This is best for him or her as well as the team and allows the individual the opportunity to depart with the least disruption to the workplace and to the individual's pride.

Hiring, reviewing, addressing performance issues, and dismissing staff are all important components of your role as a manager. Allowing behaviors or poor performance to affect the care you provide patients or interfere with a productive workplace is your responsibility as a frontline manager. The faster you intervene and the more engaged you are in the process of recognizing the issues and acting on them will gain the respect of your staff, the physicians who work in your area, and the care you provide.

PART ONE

Conclusion

Nancy Bateman

CASE STUDY

While working in a community hospital that was facing financial difficulty it became necessary to reduce staffing levels. Patient volume fell along with the town's population, and hospital leadership recognized that census figures would not increase until the town's economy improved.

Analysis was performed to determine baseline productivity, percentage of overtime, and use of agency and traveling nurses upon the start of the project. Each department was reviewed for their worked hours per unit of measure, and this was then benchmarked against similar facilities within a large database of hospitals with similar client sizes, demographics, patient services, and case-mix index. An examination of the case-mix index is available in Chapter 2.

Table I.1 represents a small sample of the generated report. Each department was reviewed using different units of measure for benchmarking—nursing units used patient days, whereas nonbedded units used metrics based on procedures. The emergency department used visit totals, whereas nonclinical areas (such as security or materials management) used adjusted discharges.

The results revealed an opportunity to reduce staffing by 87.85 full-time equivalents (FTEs) for a total savings of $4.2 million. Additional savings were also found in departments of security, dietary, and administrative support. The analysis also revealed that 1.87 FTEs were often working for weeks without patients assigned to their therapy and that the town's health department offered similar services. The final results of the analysis are shown in Table I.2.

Review of overtime as compared to total labor expenses showed that overtime costs were greater than 10% compared to the benchmark of 2%. This represented an additional $1.8 million in annual savings if overtime was reduced to benchmark levels. One of the reasons the hospital accrued high overtime costs was a policy that allowed departments to call in extra help on the morning of a work day when the census was higher than their "core staffing." Even if the person called in was a part-time employee, they were paid at either time-and-a-half or at the overtime rate. Each department determined their own core staffing, which was usually enough staff to take care of a patient in each of the unit's beds regardless of whether or not these beds were filled.

TABLE I.1
Sample of Generated Productivity Report

Cost Center #	Cost Center	FYTD 09 Total Worked Hours	Total Paid FTEs	Average Salary per FTE	Units of Measure Provided	Units of Measure Required	Units	Worked Hrs per Unit of Measure	Industry Benchmarks Top Quartile	Median	FTE Opportunity Top Quartile	Median	Labor $ Opportunity Top Quartile	Median	Questions / Notes
Inpatient Nursing															
601000	ICU	73,782	42.11	48,525	Pt Days	Patient Days	3,541	20.84	16.80	20.23	8.17	1.24	396,363	59,939	
601200	CCU	55,349	31.14	46,990	Pt Days	Patient Days	2,444	22.65	18.31	21.11	5.96	2.12	280,246	99,574	
601500	PICU	32,791	18.36	52,207	Pt Days	Patient Days	1,574	20.83	24.43	25.14	-	-	-	-	
601600	NICU	120,779	68.68	49,750	Pt Days	Patient Days	9,489	12.73	13.00	14.23	-	-	-	-	
607101	MEDICAL 11T	92,625	51.05	38,508	Pt Days	Patient Days	9,370	9.89	8.80	9.56	5.60	1.66	215,806	63,794	
607202	SURGICAL 10T	83,871	45.50	39,014	Pt Days	Patient Days	9,345	8.97	9.11	11.16	-	-	-	-	
607500	PEDIATRICS	35,580	20.75	43,348	Pt Days	Patient Days	2,660	13.37	12.54	15.51	1.29	-	56,102	-	
607600	ORTHO/SURG 9T	42,646	23.45	43,111	Pt Days	Patient Days	4,784	8.91	9.11	11.16	-	-	-	-	
607950	ACU CARDIO 7T	99,221	54.61	41,575	Pt Days	Patient Days	10,053	9.87	8.99	11.15	4.88	-	202,707	-	
607970	OBSTETRICS	66,703	38.72	42,821	Pt Days	Patient Days	9,792	6.81	6.65	7.17	0.92	-	39,300	-	
Emergency Department															
723000	EMERGENCY ROOM	88,551	48.35	41,753	Visits	Visits	33,491	2.64	2.23	2.51	7.53	2.38	314,239	99,400	
723400	TRAUMA	6,284	3.49	52,807	Calendar days	Visits	364	17.26	-	-	-	-	-	-	
Surgical Services															
702000	OPERATING ROOM	185,640	104.10	43,728	100's of min	OR Minutes	13,017	14.26	11.99	13.84	16.60	3.05	725,862	133,420	
703000	RECOVERY	29,554	16.06	49,078	100's of min.	Minutes	8,621	3.43	3.27	4.15	0.72	-	35,236	-	
Cardiac Services															
749200	CARDIOVASCULAR SVS	16,623	8.78	41,798	-	Procedures or Visits	45,827	0.36			-	-	-	-	
749210	CATHETERIZATION LAB	56,914	31.03	58,145	Procedures	Procedures or Visits	5,116	11.12			-	-	-	-	
749220	CARDIAC REHAB	3,629	1.98	59,812	-	Procedures or Visits	12,938	0.28			-	-	-	-	
749260	CARDIAC ARRHYTHMIA	157	0.11	60,615	-	Procedures or Visits	1,657	0.09			-	-	-	-	

Note: ACU, acute care unit; CCU, coronary care unit; FTE, full-time equivalent; ICU, intensive care unit; IV, intravenous; NICU, neonatal intensive care unit; PACU, post-anesthesia care unit; PICU, pediatric intensive care unit; RVU, relative value unit; SVS, services.

TABLE I.2
Labor Opportunity Roll Up

Department	FTE Reduction	Opportunity
OB – L&D	11.77	680,014
OB – Mom & baby	3.58	301,150
NICU	10.29	566,270
Peds/PICU	5.99	364,226
ICU	15.81	804,004
Medical oncology	13.07	677,912
Ortho/Surg	4.84	262,500
9T Respiratory	5.53	242,248
10T Surgical	1.10	35,890
Education	9	426,420
OR	5	236,900
Music therapy and art therapy	1.87	80,917
Total Opportunity	**87.85**	**4,678,451**
Severance		(439,258)
Net Total Opportunity		**4,239,193**

Note: FTE, full-time equivalent; ICU, intensive care unit; L&D, labor and delivery; NICU, neonatal intensive care unit; OB, obstetrics; OR, operating room; PICU, pediatric intensive care unit.

A review agency and traveler staff use revealed a high use of agency staff. The hospital did not use a structured paid time off (PTO) policy, allowing employees to acquire more than a month of vacation. Their hospital's sick leave policy also provided up to 30 days per year. Some staff members were on sick leave by calling in while taking per-diem assignments at a local academic hospital.

Upon completing the initial assessment, interviews began with each department head. These interviews determined the causes for overtime and overstaffing within selected departments. The main reason for overstaffing within the hospital was the department manager's resistance to match staffing to demand. If a department had 12 beds on the unit, they maintained a core staffing of 12 professional nurses. Historical trending revealed that only half of all available beds were ever used (except for intensive care units), indicating an average daily census of 50%.

Another issue impacting productivity was the routine of waiting until the end of a nurse's shift to document his or her notes, resulting in 30 to 60 minutes of overtime per individual.

At the assessment's conclusion it was clear that the hospital required a staffing model that would flex staff to match demand while providing a ready backup in case any unit had a sudden influx of patients, all without diminishing patient outcomes. The model had to be tested in a pilot department so the other department managers would learn the new system and become comfortable with their level of care. A new, structured acuity model was also necessary because many patients remained documented with high acuity levels up until their day of discharge. The inflated acuity levels supported, on paper, higher staffing levels resulting in overstaffed departments.

A flex staffing model was implemented in this hospital with an expanded float pool divided into skill levels. A well-structured float pool program was launched with a full-time staffing coordinator. With the expanded float pool, the staffing coordinator matched daily census figures to a reduced core staffing level. Polices were changed to institute PTO, and staff were educated on new overtime policies that encouraged note-taking at the time of service—eliminating unnecessary overtime costs. Department managers were required to approve overtime, were held accountable to the new policy, and were responsible for applying the hospital's new acuity tool. The hospital's transport unit, which was cut in lieu of freezing nursing wages, was restored.

The float pool was staffed by nurses who enjoyed the flexible hours, additional pay, and who did not require benefits. Transport and unit clerks allowed for the nonprofessional tasks to be handled by appropriately skilled staff members. Even with the additional hires, resulting labor savings of $3.8 million and the overtime savings of $1.8 million were achieved.

CONCLUSION

Increasing the productivity of labor within your department not only results in improved patient outcomes while maintaining budgets, but also better efficiency for the entire hospital. In this regard, it is important for Nurse Managers to have a thorough understanding of how to measure productivity, including use of nursing ratios, patient acuity, and flex staffing to meet demand. Management of these needs requires creating daily staffing plans that use the various staffing models; ensuring acuity is proficient and economical. As a Nurse Manager, there will be times when difficult steps must be taken to maintain high levels of quality. Following the guidelines provided will support your efforts to staff your department appropriately and provide quality patient care.

Managing Nonlabor and Supplies

Nancy Bateman and Thomas Behrens

The following chapters discuss nonlabor spending on material goods and services, often referred to as "the supply chain process." Use of value analysis teams (VAT), management of nonlabor supply and capital budgets, and the role of group purchasing organizations (GPO) are reviewed. Once familiar with the processes and responsibilities behind managing nonlabor and supply concerns, maintaining order within a department will become smoother and more enjoyable. The contracting of nonlabor supplies is described, including components and physician involvement at various levels. Both capital equipment purchase and how to interact with materials management are important in understanding the supply chain as well. Finally, inventory and its importance in maintaining efficiency is discussed.

4

Managing the Supply Chain

Nancy Bateman

Supply chain refers to the process of selecting, acquiring, distributing, and using material goods and services. There are many individuals and departments involved in a supply chain, both within and outside of an organization. Knowing how they interact and how managers can use supply chains to operate within a departmental budget are important when designing and facilitating a smoothly run, cost-effective department. Supplies and services account for 20% to 40% of a total operating budget, representing the second highest typical budgetary expense.

LEARNING OBJECTIVES

1. Define supply chain to explain how supply dollars are spent.
2. Identify health care supply chain waste and strategies for reducing it.
3. Use financial reports to track variances in spending and usage.
4. Identify factors used to evaluate new technology.
5. Define the structure of a value analysis team (VAT).
6. Identify the support roles within VAT.
7. Describe the process for new product and new technology introduction.

NONLABOR EXPENSES

Many expenses are included in the term *nonlabor*. Although most nurses only think of nonlabor expenses as patient care items, departmental budgets for supplies and nonlabor items include paper supplies, forms and contracts for linen processing, and equipment maintenance. Table 4.1 lists examples of nonlabor supplies and purchased services that are part of a supply chain budget.

The amount of products and services that fall into the nonlabor definition are broad. Even if a specific department's budget is not directly responsible for all of the

TABLE 4.1
Nonlabor Supplies and Purchased Services

Drugs, Supplies, and Consumables	Purchased Services and Other Nonlabor
Medical/surgical supplies	Repairs and maintenance
Implants	Service contracts
Films and contrasts	Medical equipment services
Drugs	Equipment rental and leases
Reagents	Utilities
Blood products	Telecommunication (pagers, phone service, cell phones)
Sutures	Reference lab testing
Instruments	Temporary labor
Valves and rings	Waste disposal
Pacers and defibrillators	Transcription
Grafts	Professional services
Balloons and stents	Memberships and dues
Gases	Printing
IV solutions and sets	External storage
Food	Travel
Linen and linen processing	
Maintenance supplies (light bulbs, batteries, HVAC)	
Office supplies	
Forms	
Books and subscriptions	

Note: IV, intravenous; HVAC, heating, ventilation, and air conditioning.

line items represented in Table 4.1, remaining on budget will still contribute to the overall viability of a facility after understanding how supply chain processes flow across an organization.

A key advantage of understanding supply chain budgeting is the opportunity for department managers to work with stakeholders to standardize products, thereby reducing redundancies and costs. This leverages the total volume of nonlabor supplies, providing support to materials management departments when negotiating pricing and terms.

SUPPLY CHAIN SPENDING

Figure 4.1 exhibits the common distribution of supply expenses at the facility level. The figure demonstrates the cost of physician preference items, accounting for the greatest budgetary spending, and displays where these items are used most frequently.

WHAT ARE THE LINKS IN THE SUPPLY CHAIN?

A supply chain can be broken down into four main links: selection, acquisition, distribution, and utilization. Discussing these links in detail demonstrates their individual importance and impact on an overall budget. A supply chain relies on these

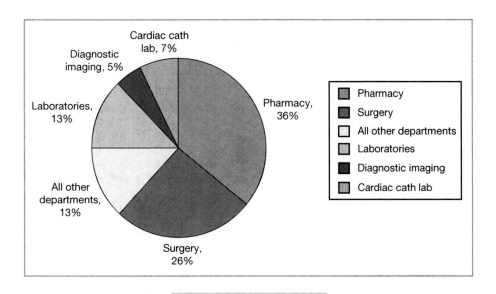

FIGURE 4.1
Distribution of Supply Expenses at Facility Level

links to drive performance and sustainability—any weakness within one section could compromise the viability of the entire chain.

Selection

Selection refers to the process by which products are requested. Because nearly 55% of supply chain costs relate to products, vendors, and efficient use of materials, clinician involvement is of the utmost importance within the selection process.

In many scenarios an intensive care unit (ICU) uses different vendors for the same products found in emergency departments (EDs) and operating rooms (ORs), increasing costs due to redundancies in suppliers. Clinicians need to discuss product selection with materials management departments to ensure that products and services are ordered through a single vendor. Being able to provide this information to materials management allows it to conduct better research and receive better bulk pricing on products. Additionally, these discussions can help control the number of vendors used within the system, increasing efficiencies throughout the other links of a supply chain.

When clinicians and physicians return from seminars and conferences, they often bring back great product ideas they wish to try. Some of the questions the materials management departments will ask are the following:

- Does this new product replace currently used products?
- Do any of our current vendors offer the same product?
- Will this new product conflict with any current contracts?
- Is the new product Food and Drug Administration (FDA) approved?
- Does the literature support the intended use of the product?
- Is this vendor contracted through our group purchasing organization (GPO)?

- What will be the usage volume of this product when negotiating price?
- How will this product be ordered and at what volume?
- Where will the product be stored?
- How dependable is the vendor for product warranty and availability?
- What orientation and training is needed?
- What capital expense is involved?

Although the process may seem complicated, materials management departments are experts in this field. Once they understand the new product and its purpose, they will work to update supply technologies and provide quality patient care while staying within budget.

Acquisition

Once products are identified and approved for purchase through a value analysis team (VAT; discussed later in this chapter), the materials management department begins with clinician involvement and acquisition. For the purposes of this chapter, the term *acquisition* applies to more than just a purchase order (PO) for products. Rather, it will incorporate sourcing, contracting, and purchasing into the acquisition link. As such, acquisition accounts for 30% of the total cost within a supply chain.

To begin the acquisition process, one must source a contract. There are many steps involved in sourcing contracts, including new products or vendors into a supply formulary (a list of commonly purchased products containing approved supply items and their substitutes based on department). Researching different vendors and their contracts is the best way to determine which vendor can provide products at the best price and with the most reliable service. Materials management departments are responsible for this work and are greatly assisted by the cooperation of clinicians. Initial research into suitable vendors begins with a hospital's GPO because these units maintain a searchable list of contracts based on vendor and product type. If current vendors can supply newly requested products, orders can be submitted faster because they have been prescreened by the hospital and reside within a materials management information system (MMIS). Once vendors are identified within an MMIS, meetings with potential vendors to discuss their products and services begin. Although these meetings are hosted by materials management departments, it is useful to include clinician input and expertise to help steer purchases.

It is important that potential vendors understand that they are not granted free access to a hospital with "a license to sell." Vendors are brought in to explain and defend the results of clinical and financial reviews of their products. Vendors are often willing to provide deep discounts on many of the items; however, it is imperative that a representative is present to determine necessary product volume. By using purchase history information, materials management departments can also provide evidence of use to support sound purchasing decisions.

Following successful clinical and financial reviews, agreements must be amended for current vendors or executed for new vendors. Amending a current agreement with a vendor is a fairly straightforward and fast process because the necessary legal and business reviews have been completed and included within the current agreement. Executing agreements with new vendors may take significantly longer. Materials management departments have agreement templates, which they edit and forward to vendors, or alternately, vendors forward agreement templates to the materials management department to begin the process. The business review of the agreement is a combined effort between materials management and the department for which the new product was ordered. Materials management will review many areas, including payment terms, shipping fees, compliance with required service levels, and the associated penalties therein. The department receiving the new product is required to review any terms regarding the successful use of the product, including training and vendor support. The main focus of a legal review is to limit the liability of an organization and to confirm that the vendor meets all regulatory and insurance requirements. Legal reviews should be requested immediately because this portion of the review can take a significant amount of time. Once a contract is completed, the item master and charge master will be updated so the buyers and accounts payable can ensure the right price is paid for the items.

Distribution

Distribution is the process of receiving, delivering, and replenishing supplies. In a well-run facility, distribution should be invisible to department staff. The old adage that "a nurse should be able to reach for the right product at the right time and in the right place" works well when communication between distribution departments is seamless. Nurse Managers are responsible for identifying products and volume requests, allowing materials management to determine suggested products and quantities based on historical usage as well as distributor and manufacturer lead times. Input from department heads is necessary when caseloads are altered and additional short-term supplies are required. Distribution and carrying costs associated with inventory represent 10% of supply chain costs, and the involvement of a Nurse Manager can impact savings in this area. Product acquisition report (PAR) levels can help demonstrate the volume of items, which should be available for use within a department. PAR may also be referred to as *min/max levels*, which refer to the minimum and maximum number of products needed in inventory at any given time. Keeping accurate trending figures for supplies helps predict future usage, helping managers alter PAR levels and order additional supplies in advance of shortages. In hospitals where automated dispensing systems are used, it is important to keep accurate software records because they are the sole metric used by materials management when ordering supplies. Finally, it is important to understand and comply with correct charging practices, as missed charges can result in lost revenue because patients will not be billed appropriately for items used during their treatment.

Understanding Distribution Methods

Understanding ordering and distribution methods is an important consideration when looking to keep supply chains operating efficiently. Different distribution methods for supplies are classified as bulk, low unit of measure (LUM), just-in-time (JIT) delivery, or STAT delivery. Their differences are explained as follows:

Bulk refers to items delivered in case quantities. With bulk ordering, it is likely that a department may receive more items than necessary because large-scale units are the only option available. Departments can avoid having to store surplus supplies by designating a central supply room or storeroom. By doing so, other departments are able to borrow additional materials as necessary.

Low unit of measure (LUM) refers to supplies ordered only in needed quantities. This option provides greater control and reduces the number of expenses riding on a department's accounts.

Just-in-time (JIT) refers to supply delivery occurring close to the time of necessity. JIT deliveries occur throughout the day, arriving in specific quantities, and can be designed to fill the needs of a department or for a particular type of clinical procedure. A clinical representative selects supplies in conjunction with the materials management department and distributes patient needs during a procedure. The supply bundle is then delivered directly to the point of need at a hospital.

STAT is similar to JIT deliveries. STAT distribution meets the immediate needs for a particular patients care. STAT deliveries are faster than JIT delivery and are more product specific. STAT also refers to small, centrally located inventories where essential supplies are always readily available.

Although LUM, JIT, and STAT deliveries are convenient, they are noticeably more expensive than bulk orders and are less efficient in the long run for many hospitals. The price for these services climbs dramatically based on the speed of delivery. As such, it is advised that hospitals make use of storerooms before other delivery services are used because storerooms allow floor staff to use bulk supplies as needed without having to find space for bulk orders on individual floors. When using storerooms, products arrive in totes marked by floor on a regular, frequent schedule, which can also boost efficiency in ways that more expensive delivery options can also provide (albeit at a greater cost). In hospitals lacking sufficient storeroom space, Nurse Managers should review the number of items needed and adjust them accordingly. In supply chain terminology, the levels of supplies are referred to as PAR levels.

Utilization

Although products can be selected carefully, priced well, and arrive in proper quantities, supply costs can still climb if ordered items are used incorrectly. Therefore, supply utilization plays a major role in a balanced budget. Waste typically accounts for 1% to 3% of supply costs. The term *waste* can refer to several factors:

Shrinkage refers to supplies that are taken home by staff, patients, and families for personal use.

Missed charges occur when patient supplies are not recorded properly, and/or charges are not properly submitted, resulting in wasted reimbursement opportunities. Missed charges can occur when automated supply cabinets are improperly kept.

Damaged goods can be unnecessary damage to supplies caused by inadequate storage locations, disposal of unused items, or soiling due to placement outside of storage.

Incorrect use of supplies are supplies that are mishandled or not used during patient care (i.e., supplies used during orientation and training that are damaged during instruction).

Understanding the supply chain is essential to managing a department. Knowing where the money is spent allows you to maintain a budget that meets patient acuity without unnecessary spending. Being able to identify waste will also result in an increased budget. The next chapter will introduce the components and processes used in creating a budget that grows.

MANAGING THE SUPPLY CHAIN BUDGET

Managing a supply chain budget requires a thorough understanding of the value analysis process (described in detail later in this chapter). Being familiar with the roles within the VAT will assist you in knowing who to go to when working with your budget. Developing the ability to calculate the factors used when evaluating new technology will ensure that your department's money is being spent effectively.

It is essential to understand budgeting practices in relation to supply chain and VAT efforts because fluency in this area will create realistic, efficient budgets, which integrate care-improving technologies.

As a Nurse Manager, one is fiscally responsible for budget management. A manager should be able to defend variances in supplies and services; by maintaining use of general ledgers (GLs), this can become a less complicated aspect of the job.

General Ledgers

Once familiar with supply budgets against actual totals, it is important to review GL subaccounts, which should be divided into major expense categories. Next, ensure that products are assigned to proper subaccounts because failure to do so can create unnecessary budget variances.

When incorrect supply items are discovered in budget subaccounts, contact the hospital's materials management department for resolution. The use of certain subaccounts throughout larger hospitals can force some items to seem out of place within their preexisting categories.

Department Budget Reviews

Many facilities conduct monthly department budget reviews, assessing supply chain costs as well as professional and overtime fees (a sample of this is shown in Figure 4.2). Specific to supply chain, managers should prepare a cost-per-case analysis for nonbedded units and a cost-per-adjusted day or cost-per-adjusted discharge analysis for supplies in bedded units.

Finance departments look at supply chain costs as a percentage of overall operations expense, supply expenses per adjusted discharge expense, and supply expenses per adjusted patient day. In this scenario, they must include the impact of outpatients in procedures as well as outpatient radiology or lab testing. This formula also takes into account overall patient acuity based on a case mix index (CMI).

When finance works with you on budgets your first step is to establish a baseline performance. Baseline metrics allow you to determine how well you are doing compared to other departments and other hospitals. Tracking monthly performance

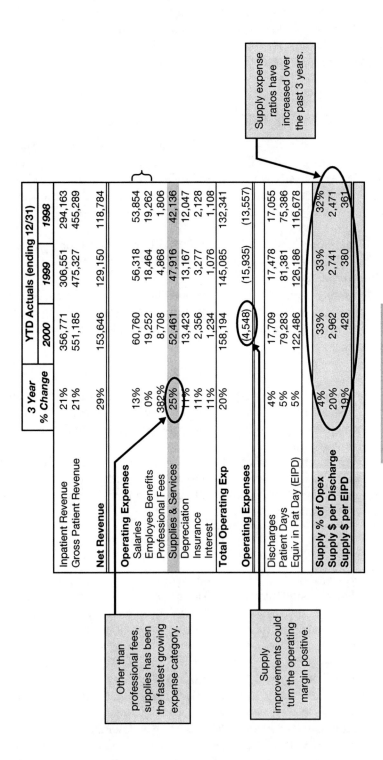

	3 Year % Change	YTD Actuals (ending 12/31)		
		2000	1999	1998
Inpatient Revenue	21%	356,771	306,551	294,163
Gross Patient Revenue	21%	551,185	475,327	455,289
Net Revenue	29%	153,646	129,150	118,784
Operating Expenses				
Salaries	13%	60,760	56,318	53,854
Employee Benefits	0%	19,252	18,464	19,262
Professional Fees	382%	8,708	4,868	1,806
Supplies & Services	25%	52,461	47,916	42,136
Depreciation	11%	13,423	13,167	12,047
Insurance	11%	2,356	3,277	2,128
Interest	11%	1,234	1,076	1,108
Total Operating Exp	20%	158,194	145,085	132,341
Operating Expenses		(4,548)	(15,935)	(13,557)
Discharges	4%	17,709	17,478	17,055
Patient Days	5%	79,283	81,381	75,386
Equiv in Pat Day (EIPD)	5%	122,486	126,186	116,678
Supply % of Opex	4%	33%	33%	32%
Supply $ per Discharge	20%	2,962	2,741	2,471
Supply $ per EIPD	19%	428	380	361

Supply expense ratios have increased over the past 3 years.

Other than professional fees, supplies has been the fastest growing expense category.

Supply improvements could turn the operating margin positive.

FIGURE 4.2
Supply Chain Costs Analysis

against your baseline helps control costs and allows for corrective action when supply costs begin to increase. Just as we compare benchmarks for productivity in quartiles, your supply cost results can also be compared by quartiles. Different from productivity calculations using worked care hours for supply costs the metrics are caculated and benchmarked against total operating costs or adjusted patient days and discharges. In areas such as the operating room you should track your supply costs per case. The simple calculation of total department supply expense divided by your total number of cases gives you a "cost per case" metric. The more global metric of supply expense as a percent of total operating costs is easy to calculate and track. When using this metric use your total operating expense minus interest, bad debt, and depreciation. This allows for a more accurate measurement.

SUPPLY COSTS AND THE IMPACT OF NEW TECHNOLOGY

The impact of new technology can increase supply costs, with expenditures outpacing normal inflation. In fact, Blue Cross Blue Shield Association commissioned a study that cited new technology as a leading cause for double-digit increases in health care costs (Kocakulah, Putman, & Vermeer, 2004).

Consumerism and Advertising Roles in Supply Costs

In addition to the costs of new technology, consumerism plays a role in the use of new devices. Consumerism is a strategy that proponents believe can improve quality of care, restrain or even reduce spending, and most importantly align attitudes and expectations of payers, providers, consumers, insurers, and the government for overall better health care outcomes. Eight of 10 Internet users have looked for health care information online, with increased interest in diet, fitness, drugs, health insurance, experimental treatments, and particular doctors and hospitals. As consumers are asked to contribute more to their health care coverage costs, they are pushing for more information and higher quality of service. In response, new forms of direct-to-consumer advertising (DTCA) within the health care industries resulted in sizeable investments over a 5-year period (1996–2000) from $600 million to $2.5 billion (Herndon, Hwang, & Bozic, 2007, p. 1294).

The Role of Advertising and Marketing in Health Care Costs

As we know, most current advertising is designed for physicians and pharmaceutical companies, although medical device manufacturers have begun targeting consumers directly. FDA-developed guidelines for the pharmaceutical industry are already in place. At the same time, similar guidelines for medical device advertising are lacking (Herndon et al., 2007, p. 1294). This can create special challenges for hospitals when evaluating new technology.

New Technology Assessment Committees

It is useful to establish a New Technology Assessment Committee (NTAC), which can control supply costs and maintain a controlled supply budget. The NTAC should be given the authority to review new technology requests, determining cost and quality benefits of the new technology within a capital budget and/or supply formulary.

Factors in the Evaluation of New Technology

- Purchase price to include maintenance costs, operating costs, and physician and staff training
- Projected revenues and reimbursement by payer
- Life expectancy of the equipment
- Risks versus clinical outcomes
- Opportunity costs
- Relevant and nonrelevant costs
- Influence costs and clinical need

Factors driving the selection and utilization of new technology within health care include clinical need as well as physician and patient requests. Clinical need is a factor when there are no technological alternatives to an available product, patient requests often stem from advertising and are not based on clinical efficacy, and physician requests result from significant involvement in acquiring processes. While purchasing new technologies for physicians can increase expenses, this can also be used to attract new doctors to a hospital (Herndon et al., 2007, p. 1294). Physician requests can be managed through the work of a VAT as explained later in this chapter.

Relevant Costs, Nonrelevant Costs, and Opportunity Costs

Relevant costs are defined as costs that differ between alternatives (such as the value of equipment being replaced by newer technology), whereas *nonrelevant costs* remain the same regardless of available alternatives (Kocakulah et al., 2004, p. 52). Decisions on new technology should only consider relevant costs.

Opportunity costs relate to forecasting, measuring the financial repercussions of not acting, so they are not usually a part of an accounting return on investment analysis. When evaluating opportunity costs, alternative courses of action should be considered and an economic value placed on each course of action. These values could represent the cost of not choosing the new technology.

Considerations When Purchasing New Technology

Equipment life expectancy should be documented in a business case to help determine replacement plans, software updates, or the acquisition of ancillary products. For all new technologies, medical–legal risks and clinical outcomes are significant components of the evaluation. New technologies can also come with risks because medical devices have been known to fail. For example, cardiac defibrillators have failed to fire or short-circuited, causing patient deaths. With the increasing costs of new technologies, payers are now requiring more stringent clinical trials prior to general release to the public. The Centers for Medicare and Medicaid Services (CMS) may not approve payment for high-risk and expensive new technologies (Herndon et al., 2007, p. 1296).

Overuse and Responsible Use of New Technology

The *moral hazard argument*, as it relates to overuse of new and expensive technology, is defined as "the responsible parties who select and use a new device . . . are not the parties responsible for the financial impact of its use" (Herndon et al., 2007, p. 1296). In order for hospitals to offer technologies to patients responsibly, it is imperative that they request clear documentation of clinical trial results and proven outcomes. New and expensive equipment must be proven worthwhile before being used on patients.

Medicare and Medicaid Reimbursement in New Technologies

Projected revenues and reimbursement by payers plays a more significant role in modern health care than ever before. As medical device prices continue to rise, hospital and physician reimbursements are not increasing at the same rate. Between 1991 and 2006, total hip implant prices rose by 171%, whereas Medicare hospital reimbursement only increased by 19%, and physician reimbursement was reduced by 13% (Herndon et al., 2007, p. 1294).

New technology is more than an enhancement to a current device. For existing vendor contracts on equipment and supplies, unless payers acknowledge the new technology with increased payments, the device is not revolutionary but evolutionary and should remain in the same cost range. Managers should make certain that purchase prices include the cost of maintenance, service contracts, operating costs, and the education of staff and physicians. The NTAC should make a final determination using a process that combines as many of these factors as possible.

FINANCIAL ANALYSIS AND COST MODELING

The standard form of financial analysis for new technology is the net present value (NPV) and/or the internal rate of return (IRR). Decision support systems specific to health care new technology were developed in 2003, looking beyond NPV and IRR to include safety, clinical features, technical features, and operating costs. Use of decision support systems account for these additional criteria, include the opinions and statistics generated by end users, and support hospitals when negotiating prices with vendors (Kocakulah et al., 2004, p. 50).

Economic modeling technologies make reviews in terms of cost-effectiveness and cost benefit as they relate to overall patient health and age, evaluating products based on adjusted life years due to the benefits of medical treatment. In 2000, the health care cost per life averaged $30,000 annually. By 2005, the health care cost per life year reached $600,000 annually. Based on these calculations, only technology related to heart attacks, cataracts, low birth weight infants, and depression demonstrated a cost benefit, which was greater than the expense of the technologies themselves (PricewaterhouseCoopers, 2005, p. 46).

An example of this cost-benefit modeling would consider the costs associated with the type of total hip components selected for a patient who is 50 years old, versus a 63-year-old and a 70-year-old. In this example, it could be determined that there is a 19% cost savings as it relates to a 20-year failure wherein a revision would be required. For the 63-year-old patient, there was a lifetime cost increase regardless of revision rate; if the cost of a high-end artificial hip was only $500 more than a standard hip, cost savings could be realized. For the 70-year-old patient, there is no scenario where cost savings would be realized. Cost-effective studies are becoming more common, but they are still relatively rare. Since 1996, only 81 studies on hip arthroplasty have included any cost-effective data (Herndon et al., 2007, p. 1302).

When creating a supply chain budget, continually review your GL to ensure you are following the value analysis process. Become familiar with the finance and materials management departments as well as any other roles within value analysis. Most important, review the factors used to evaluate new technology. Make sure your supply costs do not outpace normal inflation. Consider consumerism, advertising, and marketing costs when integrating new products into your routine.

VALUE ANALYSIS—A "SILVER BULLET" FOR SUPPLY COSTS

Value analysis can be defined as a structured process for frontline users to evaluate and make decisions regarding product selection and usage. It is important to understand the process in order to create a VAT that is efficient. The roles of VAT members should be well defined and understood. Introducing new products to your department can be a wonderful way to increase quality of care, and ensure that patient quality of care is met. Do not allow misunderstandings while analyzing value to interfere with your supply costs.

A well-structured VAT can act as a silver bullet for controlling supply costs and communicating with departments to evaluate new and current products for use within a hospital.

Roles of the Value Analysis Team Members

The major roles of the VAT are

- Evaluate all items that are used more than once
- Act as the central clearinghouse for products
- Maintain a well-defined supply formulary
- Communicate product change information
- Involve end users in new product evaluation
- Direct current product evaluation to standardize items
- Provide a venue for stakeholder involvement, feedback, and physician connectivity

The Composition of a Value Analysis Team

A VAT is composed of six layers of members, with a side layer of communication. (See Figure 4.3 for a visual representation of the VAT structure.) The top layer provides administrative support and consists of C-suite executives (CEOs, CFOs, COOs,

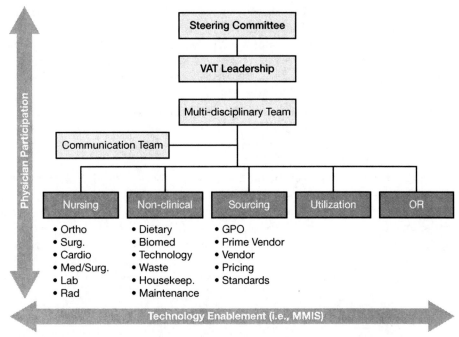

Note: OR, operating room; GPO, group purchasing organization; MMIS, materials management information system.

FIGURE 4.3
Visual Representation of the VAT Structure

CNOs, CMOs). This layer reviews monthly or quarterly reports and supports or vetoes committee decisions. C-suite members must convey decisions quickly as they affect supply orders and staff item requests.

The second VAT layer includes materials management directors, clinical analysts, and staff members. This layer of professionals reviews product requests, determines agendas, and creates review assignments for subgroups for the purpose of providing hands-on product evaluation and feedback to the VAT.

The third layer is a multidisciplinary team including representatives from each subgroup, which is the fourth layer. This third layer meets monthly and reviews product requests as well as the work of subgroups. At this level all work and communication flows in via product requests and out with decisions on the product requests.

The VAT's fourth layer consists of the aforementioned subgroups. Each subgroup is composed of representatives from every major supply user throughout the hospital. Subgroups are end users who provide vital information about a product's effectiveness and meet monthly to discuss product requests, utilization issues, and procurement practices.

The VAT's fifth layer includes ad hoc groups and smaller subgroups, which provide further evaluation of products. Ad hoc groups are responsible for physical applications of test products as directed by subgroups. This layer meets and works as necessary, pulling from the expertise of specific staff members when required. Ad hoc groups can evaluate products in one or two meetings, performing clinical trials within two weeks' time. Ad hoc recommendation deadlines should be one month or less.

The sixth and seventh layers of a VAT include physicians invited to attend subgroup or multidisciplinary meetings as well as representatives from information systems (IS) departments. Participants in this layer are also called in as needed, depending on the product under consideration.

The communication layer is considered separate to those described earlier because of its importance across all other layers. A standing communication team should produce newsletters, poster displays, and scheduled e-mail alerts to keep staff updated on product changes.

Figure 4.4 demonstrates each step in the VAT process, identifying responsible parties in the progression of product introduction and approval.

VAT teams need to respond to requests within a two-month time frame in order to be sustainable. Although many facilities currently have VATs in place, they are not always fully represented by various departments. Many VAT are too slow to respond and do not look at multiple requests at once. This leads to outside staff undermining VAT processes, as well as general decision-making slowdowns.

Value Analysis Team Decisions in Urgent Care

In a well-structured VAT there are policies in place for urgently needed supplies. The following is a guideline for defining urgent requests:

- Life-threatening situations
- Urgent/emergent surgical procedures
- Patient-specific needs
- Loss of efficiency

Once an urgent request policy is implemented it should be monitored carefully for staff and physician compliance.

Measuring Value Analysis Team Value and Efficacy

Ultimately, VAT activities will need to be tracked to demonstrate their effectiveness. Teams must be able to report savings and standardization achievements gained through the process. The use of a dashboard can help report baseline levels (pre-VAT assessments), target levels (projected accomplishments), and monthly/quarterly results. VAT should assess their program's usefulness with the following criteria.

Effective Performance Measures
- Frequency/volume of urgent requests
- Provision of feedback to requestors within one week of VAT decision
- Decrease in nonfiled requests
- Departments should meet supply budget
- Information to be submitted to VAT within two weeks of original request
- Achieve success in savings

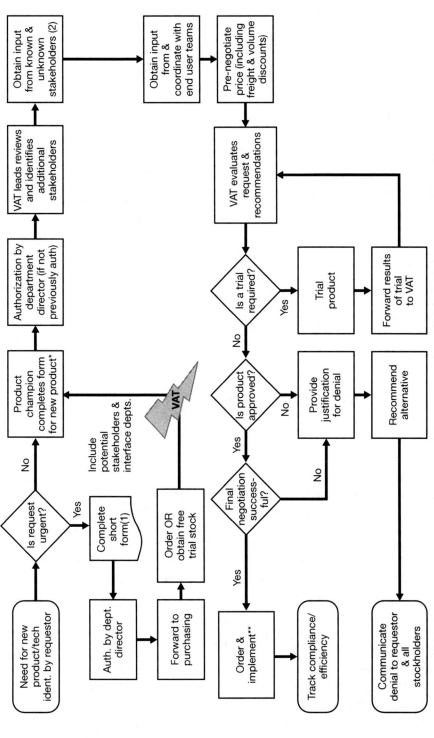

FIGURE 4.4
New Product Request Process

Note: *New Product Request form will include information on savings potential, stakeholders, and interfacing departments.
**Implementation includes training, stocking, converting old product, vendor negotiations, communication, and changes in information systems (IS).
(1) Limit of **$10,000** for clinical products and **$1,000** for non-clinical products.
(2) Includes managed care, finance, and risk management.

59

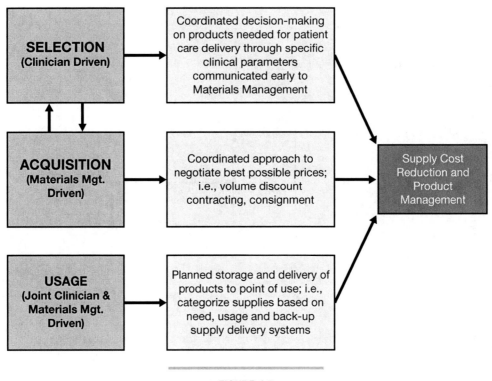

FIGURE 4.5
Approach to Product Management

When clinicians and materials management directors can work together to provide the right products for each department at the best prices, VAT processes can provide a cost benefit to a hospital. Figure 4.5 shows how supply cost can be reduced by using this approach to product management. Figure 4.5 demonstrates clinicians ordering products based on demand, regardless of existing vendor relationships. By ordering products based on use, instead of by vendor, new products and suppliers can enter the acquisition picture. While this can contribute to increasing supply costs, it also provides new materials for improving care.

Product Evaluation

There are specific guiding principles one should consider when evaluating any new product. A sample evaluation form and evaluation criteria can be found within the VAT Toolkit in Appendix B. The process is very involved, although setting up or revamping current processes is well worth the time and effort required. Remember to track the successes of the VAT because this should be reported to the finance department when making budgetary decisions. Steps within the VAT Toolkit, shown in the following section, can be used in whole or in part—creating new VATs or filling gaps in preexisting systems.

VALUE ANALYSIS TEAM TOOLKIT

Section I

A. Purpose and Objectives of Value Analysis
Purpose
Value analysis reduces nonlabor expenses while providing quality products to [HOSPITAL NAME] in a competitive, cost-conscious market. The ultimate goal of the value analysis process is to provide facility flexibility while optimizing the hospital's buying power. This is achieved through the creation of a structure, which focuses on better product utilization, standardization, and the management of new products and technology.

Objectives
- Provide a strong value analysis team (VAT) framework
- Define job roles and responsibilities of VAT leaders
- Define job roles and responsibilities of VAT members
- Communicate product utilization guidelines
- Communicate organizational sales representative policies
- Increase employee and physician awareness and accountability for better management of supply costs
- Assure timely, consistent product trial and evaluation processes
- Decrease product expenditures by selecting effective and economical products based on trials and evaluations
- Monitor and measure product usage and expenditures
- Monitor company-wide product usage

B. Guiding Principles for the Value Analysis Process
The following principles will be used during the value analysis process to analyze product need, cost, utilization, and ability to support quality service.

Quality
Quality is a composite criterion emphasizing performance, including an item's durability, reliability, integrity, and benefits to care delivery.

EXAMPLE: How durable is a pair of gloves during normal use? How often do the gloves tear?

Effectiveness
Effectiveness is a measurement of an item's ability to meet its intended purpose.

EXAMPLE: Do a pair of gloves meet its intended function? How well do the gloves protect one's hands? Do the gloves allow for sufficient tactile response?

Cost
Costs include acquisition, holding, stocking, handling, disposal, and processing expenses. Product utilization is another aspect of cost, which includes frequency of use and the selection of appropriate products and devices.

EXAMPLE: Are all the benefits worth the price?

Storage/Space Availability
Storage space and requirements will be considered.

EXAMPLE: Is there sufficient storage space for the item?

Packaging
Optimal packaging will have minimal waste and ease of opening.

EXAMPLE: Is the item packaged as desired? Does the item require any special tools or methods for opening its packaging? Is there unnecessary waste with the packaging?

Availability
The product must be available when needed.

EXAMPLE: Are there adequate options available concerning the acquisition or distribution of this item?

Operation
Consider the impact of using the product and compatibility within a current system.

EXAMPLE: Will the item require forceful, frequent, repetitive motions with operation? Is the item difficult or awkward to use?

Education/Training
Consider education and training requirements.

EXAMPLE: Does the item require any special training for use? Does this item require training for compliance with regulatory requirements? Who will be responsible for providing training?

Safety/Infection Control/Waste Management
The item will comply with all hospital, The Joint Commission (TJC), and Occupational Safety and Health Administration (OSHA) regulations/requirements.

EXAMPLE: Is there an increased risk of injury (i.e., sharps injury or back injury)? If the item is disposable, does it have any special disposal requirements? If the item is reusable, does it require any special reprocessing? Is the product invasive? Does the product come into contact with nonintact skin or mucous membrane?

Service and Repair
Vendor provision of service and repair time will meet the user's need.

EXAMPLE: Can an item be repaired in-house? Are preventative maintenance agreements needed?

SECTION II

Roles and Working Relationships

A. Value Analysis Steering Committee
Scope
The purpose of the committee is to establish and monitor a process for timely, cost-effective, and value-oriented product acquisition across the organization. It will develop ongoing performance measures at each level of the team structure.

Responsibilities
- Ensures that value analysis procedures are maintained
- Reviews product team decisions to ensure that guiding principles are used when selecting items
- Challenges product team decisions if guiding principles were not followed
- Develops ongoing measurement tools to advance the work of the VAT
- Resolves conflicts regarding product use when consensus cannot be reached
- Ensures accurate documentation regarding product cost savings and team accomplishments
- Provides final approval of all products following team decisions
- Establishes monthly committee meetings
- Serves a 2-year term

Value Analysis Steering Committee Roles and Responsibilities

B. Vice President Materials Management
- Responsible for value analysis processes and supply chain activities throughout the hospital
- Reports contractual updates supplied by the VAT
- Facilitates in development of performance tracking measures for each of the team structures
- Empowers and integrates the value analysis process with clinical/operational structures to achieve measurable outcomes
- Chairs the Value Analysis Steering Committee
- Communicates system budget adjustments resulting from cost savings
- Approves policies and/or procedures in relation to product use standardization
- Makes decisions regarding product selection when VAT cannot reach consensus

C. Value Analysis Manager/Coordinator
- Reviews and revises product use standardization procedures in conjunction with the VAT
- Develops steering committee meeting agendas
- Facilitates and monitors all VAT activities
- Evaluates and prioritizes opportunities for usage standardization within logistics, finance, and operations departments as well as through discussions with administrators, physicians, and staff
- Cochairs with VAT team lead, coordinate subcommittee and ad hoc meetings
- Manages and provides value analysis information by maintaining a cost-saving tracking system
- Coordinates efforts with the biomedical equipment department to optimize supply equipment contracts
- Analyzes follow-up reports to determine effectiveness of current efforts
- Evaluates annual performance of VAT members based on established team member responsibilities

- Interacts with patient care staff to receive feedback before making product decisions
- Interacts with applicable departments to address safety, regulatory, and epidemiology issues prior to product selection
- Collaborates with others to develop and implement monitoring plans for product standardization
- Coordinates educational activities related to product use
- Uses product selection guidelines to evaluate product requests
- Streamlines product entry processes with adherence to established time lines
- Develops annual goals and objectives with VAT members
- Analyzes cost-savings ideas and implement standardization opportunities
- Reports to the Value Analysis Steering Committee

D. Value Analysis Steering Committee Member (Includes Financial and Materials Members)

- Reviews product team decisions, ensuring that value analysis process guiding principles were used during product selection
- Ensures that staff and physician education was conducted prior to product use
- Ensures accurate documentation is available regarding product cost savings and team accomplishments
- Participates in team meetings, attending a minimum of 75% of yearly meetings
- Adheres to meeting ground rules
- Performs assignments in a timely and accurate manner
- Reports outcomes to the Value Analysis Steering Committee

Value Analysis Team

Scope
The purpose of the team is to design and implement product decisions based on steering committee recommendations and the guiding principles of the value analysis process.

Responsibilities
- Analyzes, evaluates, and monitors all trials, selecting the most cost-effective product for use
- Investigates and removes product redundancies
- Reviews product usage for economic impact
- Ensures benchmarking and/or literature reviews are completed prior to product selection
- Enlists experts and/or end users to assist in product evaluation
- Ensures maintenance of the value analysis process
- Performs group purchasing organization (GPO) product validations
- Coordinates product implementation and education
- Reports product recommendations and decisions to Value Analysis Steering Committee for review
- Meets monthly to review new projects and objectives
- Serves a 2-year term

Value Analysis Team Roles and Responsibilities

Team Leader

- This position is also a team member for the Steering Committee
- Develops meeting agendas, conducts team meetings, and records meeting minutes
- Provides direction and focus for team activities
- Ensures productive use of team members' time
- Reports team progress to the Value Analysis Steering Committee
- Documents team activities and outcomes; assess team progress
- Encourages and promotes creative problem solving
- Advocates and becomes a sponsor of change
- Makes decisions related to team member performance
- Ensures usage of "Guiding Principles for Value Analysis Process" during product selection
- Ensures education requirements are completed before a new product is placed in use
- Facilitates ongoing policy and procedure reviews for usage standardization

E. Materials Manager Value Analysis Team Member

- Investigates and reports contractual obligations regarding proposed changes prior to proposal generation
- Performs and provides software system research as needed or requested (i.e., historical product usage by department)
- Obtains product information (item description, catalog number, vendor or supplier, order quantity, and pricing)
- Prepares value analysis reports for team recommendation/decision making
- Obtains samples when needed for education sessions
- Determines stocking for approved products with logistic services personnel
- Collaborates with the value analysis manager/coordinator, adding new products to existing supply contracts or establishing new supply contracts
- Collaborates with materials management personnel and/or external suppliers to ensure adequate stock is available and provided to departments
- Plans for return and/or use of existing product inventory before initiating product changes
- Supplies new product item numbers and implementation target dates
- Provides the value analysis manager/coordinator with proposed and actual implementation dates
- Provides cost center budget adjustment data with supporting documentation
- Directs material management/purchasing to discontinue multiple products after deciding to use single products

F. Value Analysis Team Member

- Offers personal perspective and ideas
- Participates actively in a minimum of 75% of team meetings

- Adheres to meeting ground rules
- Performs assignments accurately and in a timely manner
- Supports implementation of approved recommendations
- Confers with colleagues to understand issues arising from product changes
- Considers the impact of selecting new products on quality patient services and value analysis
- Represents the majority of coworkers when making product decisions
- Maintains objectivity when selecting new products
- Advocates change and propose new ideas

G. Value Analysis Product Champion (May Also Be a Physician)

- Identifies and contacts product end users to determine common usage, practice changes, and average costs
- Maintains vendor price confidentiality
- Provides literature and hospital benchmarking regarding product use when appropriate
- Identifies educational requirements and ensure completion before the product is placed in use

In summary, Table 4.2 is a start-up checklist that will help pull it all together.

TABLE 4.2
Value Analysis Start-Up Checklist

Topic	What Is Expected	Helpful Materials/Items
Material director's conference call	– Question and answer related to start up process for value analysis – Define materials director's roles and responsibilities	– Value Analysis Team Start-Up Checklist – Value Analysis Team Toolkit – Drafts of advisory council team charters
Value analysis team leaders and team members	– Select team leader and four to six team members for local surgical services team – Select team leader and four to six team members for local cardiac cath/diagnostic imaging team – Identify contact for surgical services and cardiac cath/diagnostic imaging, if currently performing value analysis – E-mail the aforementioned information to national director of contracting and value analysis	– Team leader roles and responsibilities document from Value Analysis Team Toolkit (Appendix B) – Team member roles and responsibilities document from Value Analysis Team Toolkit (Appendix B) – Sample job descriptions from Value Analysis Team Toolkit (Appendix B)

(continued)

TABLE 4.2 *(continued)*

Value Analysis Start-Up Checklist

Topic	What Is Expected	Helpful Materials/Items
Value Analysis Communication Toolkit	– Review Value Analysis Communication Toolkit	– Value Analysis Communication Toolkit
Material director's and/or supply chain sponsor meet with selected team leaders	– Review roles and responsibilities – Provide value analysis materials that have been received to date	– Value Analysis Team Toolkit – Value Analysis Team Start-Up Checklist – Drafts of advisory council team charters – Value Analysis Communication Toolkit
Supply chain sponsor call	– Supply chain sponsor update on value analysis rollout plans – Solicit feedback	– All materials received to date
Team leader orientation videoconferences	– Local value analysis team leaders for surgical services and cardiac cath/diagnostic imaging will attend one of the three available orientation videoconferences – Materials director and supply chain sponsor	– All materials received to date
Value analysis schedule is defined	– Meetings to be held at least monthly, closely following enclosed schedule (if not, please set schedule for next 12 months) – Materials director and team leader determine schedule and submit for the surgical services and cardiac cath/diagnostic imaging value analysis teams	– Proposed meeting schedule January 1-4 February 4-8 March 4-8 April 1-5 May 1–3 June 3-7 July 1-5 August 5-9 September 2-6 October 1-4 November 4-8 December 2-6
Value analysis teams are chartered	– Materials director and value analysis team leaders will complete team charters	– Draft advisory council team charters
Kickoff/initial value analysis meetings	– Materials director and value analysis team leaders will conduct initial meetings	– Proposed agenda in Value Analysis Team Toolkit (Appendix B)
Status reporting	– Materials director and value analysis team leaders complete status report for each team	– Work plan/status report in Value Analysis Team Toolkit (Appendix B)
Ongoing value analysis meetings	– Materials director and value analysis team leader will gather product information to support teamwork and review	– Prioritized initiatives from advisory councils – Local contracting initiatives requiring value analysis input

Once a structure is in place, include representatives from infection control, education, and biomedical departments as they can contribute to the successful launch of new products by presenting perspective, providing training and orientation support, reporting effects on quality, and reporting any necessary biomedical requirements.

SUMMARY

In order to provide facility flexibility while optimizing the hospital's buying power, which is the ultimate goal for value analysis, it is essential to be comfortable with the entire process. The roles within your value analysis team go beyond the six layers, with a side layer of communication to ensure that funds are being spent appropriately. The introduction of new materials that enhance patient quality of care must be monitored closely. Follow the "New Product Request Process" to make sure that parties are responsible for their roles while progressing from new product introduction to approval. See the sample evaluation form in Appendix B of this textbook for further assistance when purchasing new products.

5

Strategies for Achieving Cost Effectiveness

Nancy Bateman, Gregg Lambert, and Marilyn Connell

A group purchasing organization (GPO) may be used to provide value while purchasing new products for your department. This organization will assist you in contracting for supplies, services, and capital equipment. It is important to understand the role of a GPO and how to use a group purchasing contract when acquiring new materials. As such, this chapter will explain the difference between a sole source agreement and a multisource agreement. It will also help you when working with companies that already have a contract in place versus setting up a new relationship with a different company and a new contract. The various contract tiers are described to assist you in obtaining the best possible price for your budget.

LEARNING OBJECTIVES

1. Define group purchasing organizations (GPO) and explain how they relate to supply contracting.
2. Use GPO contracts as a tool.
3. Understand GPO contract tier and when to work with your supply chain team to increase tier levels on select product categories.
4. Identify the data components of contracts required for effective contracting.
5. Understand the importance of physician involvement.
6. Define capital equipment and articulate the purchase process.
7. List components of a complete capital equipment request for materials management.
8. List components of inventory management.
9. Identify and work with the inventory type used in your department.
10. Define physical inventory and participate in the process.

GROUP PURCHASING ORGANIZATIONS

A facility's use of their GPO plays an important role in nonlabor supply chain considerations. Many facilities are members of GPOs, which provide many benefits including the following:

- GPOs work with many hospitals to leverage buying power to achieve lower prices and better contract terms for medical supplies, services, and capital equipment for their members.
- GPOs offer favorable pricing on goods, services, and capital equipment, influencing suppliers to keep market prices lower.
- GPOs collect administrative fees from vendors, based on sales, that finance their operations. This allows GPOs to deliver patronage dividends, shareholder distributions, and value-added services to the members.

GPOs negotiate contracts with vendors on behalf of members, approaching multiple vendors with the accumulated purchasing volume of their members as leverage for pricing and contract-term negotiation. Within a GPO, members can achieve different pricing levels (tiers) based on their purchasing habits. Contracts are set up with tiered pricing to encourage standardization and use of the GPO contracts. Higher purchase percentages translate to higher tiers with vendors lowering overall prices.

Working With Group Purchasing Organizations

The largest GPOs are Novation, Premier, HealthTrust, Amerinet, and MedAssets, which operate similarly while requiring varying degrees of commitment. It is important to understand how a hospital's GPO works because new product introduction and selection should be done in accordance with purchasing options and policies. GPOs have differing methods for providing value in terms of contracting for supplies, services, and capital equipment. Some offer membership a broad-ranging contract portfolio that encompasses a large percentage of a hospital's needs. Others have a less complete portfolio and partner with a hospital or Integrated Delivery Network (IDN—a hospital-based system for acquiring supplies outside of a GPO) to put agreements into place on a custom, hospital-based level.

Understanding Group Purchasing Organization Contracts

GPOs differ in their philosophies on compliance to their contracts. As a general rule, vendors reward higher compliance with lower pricing and better contract terms. Penalties for noncompliance range from written or verbal communication to potential rejection from a GPO. Buying products or services off-contract can negatively impact a facility, exposing it to higher product prices. Speak with a materials management director to understand more about GPO compliance. Whether a hospital belongs to a highly compliant GPO or not, one should become familiar with its GPO contract portfolio. As needs arise for supplies, services, or capital equipment, GPOs provide sourcing solutions whether or not a current contract is in place. When contracts are in place, receiving products is as simple as submitting orders. When no contract is in place, however, one must be created using the protocol explained earlier in this chapter.

TABLE 5.1
Multivendor Group Purchasing Organization Agreement

Vendor A			Vendor B			Vendor C		
Tier	Compliance	Price	Tier	Compliance	Price	Tier	Compliance	Price
Tier 1	90%–100%	$10.00	Tier 1	90%–100%	$11.00	Tier 1	90%–100%	$12.00
Tier 2	80%–89%	$11.00	Tier 2	80%–89%	$12.00	Tier 2	80%–89%	$13.00
Tier 3	<80%	$12.00	Tier 3	<80%	$13.00	Tier 3	<80%	$14.00

Group Purchasing Organization Contracts by Type

GPOs offer different contracts based on factors such as member input, supply, service or equipment type, or market availability. For commodity products, it is common to offer a committed or sole source agreement. In this type of agreement, a GPO has negotiated with the vendor based on the cumulative volume of the membership, and it is expected that the hospital will use the product or service to fill its needs.

Another type of GPO contract is a multisource agreement. In these circumstances, two or more vendors are awarded an agreement for identical or similar product lines and services. This contract recognizes the competitive nature of the vendors in certain product categories, allowing members to choose which available option works best for their needs. The concept of tier pricing discussed earlier is relevant when using multisource agreements because vendors reward a higher level of commitment with better pricing. Allowing physicians and staff to purchase from multiple vendors (as opposed to one of the provided, agreed-upon options) will deliver suboptimal pricing, and also cause other inefficiencies such as an increased need for storage space to house similar products from multiple vendors. Approaching materials management, physicians, and staff to choose a single vendor among the competitive offers, however, will deliver favorable pricing.

Tables 5.1 through Table 5.4 provide a scenario in which a hospital's GPO has entered into a multivendor agreement for a particular product involving three vendors. The pricing for each vendor, each tier, and each respective compliance level is shown at the top of Table 5.1. In this example, Tier 1 provides the best pricing level. This example delivers the best pricing level and may be the preferred tier in most cases. In this example, the annual usage of the contracted product is 1,000 units.

TABLE 5.2
Unmanaged Agreement Scenario

Vendor	Compliance	Price	Usage	Cost
A	35%	$12.00	350	$4,200.00
B	25%	$13.00	250	$3,250.00
C	40%	$14.00	400	$5,600.00
		Spend		$13,050.00

TABLE 5.3
Intermediate Agreement Management Scenario

Vendor	Compliance	Price	Usage	Cost		
A	10%	$12.00	100	$1,200.00		
B	80%	$12.00	800	$9,600.00		
C	10%	$14.00	100	$1,400.00	Savings	Savings (%)
		Spend		$12,200.00	$850.00	6.5

In the Unmanaged Agreement Scenario (Table 5.2), physicians and clinicians are not informed of the multiple agreements available, and are not involved in value analysis. As a result, usage and compliance are spread across all three vendors, resulting in higher prices.

In the Intermediate Agreement Management Scenario (Table 5.3), physicians and clinicians are involved in the value analysis process, resulting in an 80% compliance level with Vendor B—returning a better price for the product in return. The gains from the time and effort involved in the process is $850 ($13,050–$12,200) or 6.5% savings to a hospital's budget.

In the Optimal Agreement example (Table 5.4), an advanced education and value analysis program resulted in a 90% compliance level, with Vendor A achieving access to Tier 1 pricing. In this example, Vendor A offers the best pricing of the three vendors, so this is truly an optimized agreement scenario. Efforts in this example resulted in a savings of $2,750 ($13,050–$10,300) or 21.1% budget savings when compared with the Unmanaged Agreement Scenario.

Understanding the tiers and how to work with group purchasing is essential when contracting for new materials. GPOs will work with you to find the supplies you need at the best price. They will help you set up contracts for services and capital equipment with new businesses and facilitate the purchasing of these products with established vendors already under contract. GPOs will help you lower costs without compromising value within your department.

SUPPLY CHAIN CONTRACTING

Supply chain contracting is not just a component of the acquisition link, it is also a part of strategic sourcing, utilization management, patient demand factors, and

TABLE 5.4
Optimized Agreement Management Scenario

Vendor	Compliance	Price	Usage	Cost		
A	90%	$10.00	900	$9,000.00		
B	10%	$13.00	100	$1,300.00		
C	0%	$14.00	0	$0.00	Savings	Savings (%)
		Spend		$10,300.00	$2,750.00	21.1

clinical outcomes—all of which determine value and total cost when purchasing and incorporating new technologies. Possessing a solid understanding of the components of supply chain contracting will make the purchasing process easier for the Nurse Manager. Involving physicians in this activity is instrumental in contributing to the success of this process along with delegating roles and responsibilities as appropriate to ensure a productive and efficient working environment.

Precontract Considerations

Clinical oversight is needed to help ensure that selected products provide desired patient care outcomes: less-expensive products can still drive high overall costs if usage is not monitored, making documentation important as it maintains product efficiency and effectiveness. Value analysis and clinical integration processes, therefore, are keys to product selection, which leads to the contracting process.

Negotiating Contracts

Some hospitals implement a contracting model, which combines GPO and hospital-brokered contracts. To negotiate good contracts, it is essential to maintain current and accurate data. Data components include the following:

- Manufacturer name standardization
- Product reorder number standardization
- Product descriptive field(s) standardization
- Price
- Unit of measure (UOM) conversions (i.e., 10 to a box)
- Unit of purchase (UOP) conversions
- Cost accounting information
- Contracts
- Bin locations

Clinician and Physician Involvement in Contracting

Clinicians should engage in product selection processes from the beginning and should remain aware that materials management are looking to purchase products that provides the greatest patient value at the best price. When value analysis programs were implemented, clinicians often believed that materials management wanted to buy the lowest priced products without their consultation or evaluation. A collaborative model between materials management and clinicians must be established so that each party understands the needs of the other.

Physician support can be improved by

- Using accurate data and metrics
- Having physicians as value analysis team (VAT) members
- Promoting transparency in supply issues

Initiating Contracts

Most hospitals will develop contract templates that have been approved by legal departments or outside law counsels. Many legal agreements include the following items:

- Pricing
- Term of contract
- Payment terms
- State of legal jurisdiction

Once a hospital and a vendor have negotiated and approved the contract, a monitoring process should track compliance and savings when applicable. A monitoring process should do the following:

- Use a hospital contracting template with standard terms and conditions
- Use benchmarking services to identify and negotiate best pricing
- Control vendor visits in a facility/department
- Implement a value analysis team
- Confirm all orders to ensure accurate contract pricing
- Identify and challenge all price increases
- Convert products and services to lower cost options; institute clinically acceptable alternatives
- Standardize request for proposal (RFP) and bid processes
- Enforce existing policies and procedures
- Limit the number of employees' authority to commit hospital funds
- Track and report savings
- Hold department managers accountable for supply budgets
- Implement approval levels for departmental purchases
- Reuse and reprocess material when possible
- Standardize a medical/surgical formulary (similar to a drug formulary)
- Take advantage of desktop delivery for office products
- Use procurement cards for nonmedical high-volume, low-value items like office supplies and local maintenance items

Areas that are not normally contracted through the GPO but should be reviewed by materials management for potential standardization and cost savings include the following:

- Support services
- Travel
- Transcription
- Laundry/linen

- Waste removal
- Printing
- Shredding
- Document/records storage
- Temporary labor
- Environmental services
- Waste removal
- Vending
- Catering
- Biomedical
- Nutrition services
- Advertising/marketing
- Valet
- Landscaping/grounds maintenance
- Office supplies
- Cleaning supplies
- IT (information technology) supplies/software
- Chemicals
- Telecommunications
- Minor equipment

Development of the New Technology Assessment Committee

"Technology assessment and VATs have the potential to help hospitals improve quality of care and cost-effectiveness—if they are set up right" (Skorup, 2008, p. 96).

Hospitals face tough decisions required to reduce physician preference items, improve clinical outcomes, and provide safe and effective care. The use of VAT and New Technology Assessment Committees (NTAC; ancillary committees focused on new technology), has proven that supply spending can be controlled and even reduced while maintaining quality care. NTAC membership should include the chief finance officer, director of materials management, education department representation, biomedical engineering, risk management, ancillary departments, and nursing. Specific decision criteria, including many of the factors listed in this chapter, should be developed so that all new technology receives the same scrutiny and ensures that committee members do not make biased decisions. Clear documentation of the decision-making process is important, especially when a physician or requestor must have a request denied.

Implementation of a well-structured and evidence-based NTAC can assess the benefits, risks, and costs associated with the acquisition and use of new technologies. NTACs can provide critical assessments before new products are purchased and implemented, supporting a balance between expanded treatments and budget constraints.

Effective Contracting

To manage an effective contracting and supply chain department, the supply chain leader must do the following:

- Enforce purchasing policies/procedures
- Optimize inventory management
- Manage facility contract procedures
- Collaborate with physician/clinical staff
- Track outcomes
- Integrate systems
- Enable technology
- Use the United Nations Standard Products and Services Code (UNSPSC; a nonproprietary code system to codify goods and services), Universal Product Number (UPN) data standards

Obtaining Capital Equipment Online

Although hospitals can procure products at competitive rates using GPOs, there are various options for buying capital equipment online. Two common options are as follows:

- **eSourcing**—eSourcing is defined as the electronic procurement of products. Although purchasing have been computerized for decades, eSourcing implies more automatic procedures; especially dealing with contracts and processes that continue to be reviewed and managed entirely by individuals.
- **eAuctions**—An online opportunity to optimize the prices for products and services. eAuctions is an environment where current or prospective sellers can bid for a hospital's business. The process is controlled by the hospital and is subject to the rules developed and agreed upon before the auction's launch. Hospitals are then able to accept bids at will, buying items at competitive rates.

Acquiring new technology, services, and capital equipment requires negotiating contracts that work for your department's budget. Looking closely at all the data components throughout the process will provide essential information to assist you with negotiations. Finally, know when and how to involve physicians and clinicians from precontract considerations to the final draft.

CAPITAL EQUIPMENT EXPENDITURES

While introducing new products into your routine, it is important to consider capital equipment as a major item in your budget and your department's spending. The process of obtaining capital equipment can either fall under a ground-up or top-down methodology, and it is essential to know which method works best for you. When purchasing capital equipment, knowing what your materials management department needs for requests will help things progress smoothly from initial pricing to the printing of the receipt.

Capital equipment is a designation given to more expensive items, usually defined as costing $1,000 or more per ordering unit. These products cannot be purchased using operating and supply budgets; rather, they must be approved separately as these expenditures are monitored separately within budgeting offices. Each department or operating area submits their capital budget request to varying levels of management for approval. Eventually, a senior-level management group or individual will have the responsibility of reviewing the entire capital budget request. He or she will consider the overall capital expenditure target, strategy, and all historical spending per department or area, making final decisions or sending budget requests back to their originating parties. Taking advantage of all available sources in the hospital's capital budgeting process allows the best preparation, and therefore increases the opportunity that a project will be approved and implemented.

Capital Budgets and Approval Processes

The capital budget and approval process varies for each organization, although most hospitals employ a "ground-up" or "top-down" methodology.

The Ground-Up Budget Process—In a ground-up budget process the budget process originates at the department level. Department personnel put together a listing of desired equipment based on various inputs including staff, physician, management, and biomedical engineering. Staff is aware of equipment needs based on availability and quality. Department management shares the awareness of the staff, and may also be aware of pending strategy moves by hospital leadership such as adding a new clinical service, which will require the addition of capital equipment. In a ground-up budget model having information on the quality of current items is essential. Nurse Managers should contact biomedical engineering departments to ascertain the status of current equipment, including the frequency of repairs.

The Top-Down Budget Process—In a top-down capital budget process, senior management allocates capital funding and forwards details to department directors. Some facilities, in turn, request proposals for capital purchases after deciding allocation, requiring departments to communicate their spending plans to management.

After receiving capital project approval (when necessary), Nurse Managers should work with materials management to develop purchasing plans. The materials management department can obtain pricing information, research new models that have been available since the request was first submitted, coordinate installation plans with other departments, negotiate price and servicing plans with vendors, and file purchase orders (PO). Once orders are received, materials management oversees the receipt process, working with finance to establish new products as fixed assets. Additionally, the department will coordinate with IT and biomedical engineering to establish maintenance plans, scheduled repairs, and initial inspection.

Obtaining capital equipment is not intimidating once you understand the process and necessary materials. Being comfortable with either the ground-up or top-down methods will make acquiring technology for your department simple. Be sure your materials management department is provided with what it needs for pricing, research, installation, and service plans so it can file a purchase order that meets everyone's needs.

INVENTORY MANAGEMENT

Inventory management refers to the tracking and management of material, stockroom locations, inventory balance reconciliation, replenishment of supplies, selective inventory control, lot tracking, and the monitoring of expiration dates. As a Nurse Manager, you play an important role in inventory management working with materials management to monitor the levels of supplies stored in your department. Inventory levels directly impact cash flow in a hospital. Money tied up in supplies sitting on shelves needs to be monitored as efficiently as possible.

Components included in inventory management are as follows:

- Establishing lead time from vendors
- Carrying cost of inventory—the cost of taxes, insurance, and physical costs involved in storing inventory
- Asset management—tracking the location of materials and their usability
- Inventory forecasting—estimating the necessary quantity of a product or service
- Inventory valuation—a monetary value for items that make up an inventory
- Physical inventory—determining the quantity of inventory on hand through an inventory count
- Replenishment—resupplying used inventory stock
- Expiration dating—assessing and removing items past their usage date
- Returns and defective products—sending unneeded or defective items back to vendors

Areas that impact inventory management include the following:

- Unofficial inventories found throughout the facility that can account for as much as 50% of total inventories
- Accurate, real-time information systems with interfaces to appropriate financial and clinical systems
- Support from clinical and other internal customers

Materials management can deliver significant improvements to optimize the workflows and processes associated with a hospital's Materials Management Information System (MMIS), thus reducing inventory-related costs. These improvements include cost reduction opportunities for items beyond the scope of inventory. Case studies have shown the following results:

- A 5% to 20% reduction in inventory investment in the first year
- A 5% to 10% reduction in supply spent over 2 years
- Lower overnight freight costs
- Optimized inventory levels

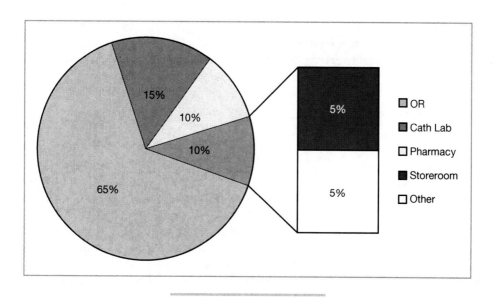

FIGURE 5.1
Clinical Inventories

- Identification of products for inclusion in an item master
- Identify PAR (order point) levels based on usage
- Improved patient care and safety
- Increased identification of expired product
- Increased efficiencies
- Improved focus on patient care
- Elimination of redundant work
- Increased use of automated IT processes

Clinical inventories usually represent 80% of the total hospital inventory value as shown in Figure 5.1. Looking at the figure, there is 65% housed in the operating rooms (OR) and 15% in the cath labs. The remaining inventory sits in pharmacy (10%), the storeroom (5%), and the final 5% is the supplies stored across all other departments. Figure 5.1 is divided by spend versus the number of supplies. One of the reasons that expenditure is highest in the OR and cath lab is because of the high dollar technology and physician preference supplies.

Inventory Classification

Hospitals normally treat inventory in one of two ways as shown in the following:

1. **Expensed upon receipt**: Products are expensed to ordering departments upon receipt at the hospital. Products are ordered and received into the warehouse, but are also immediately charged to a departmental budget.

2. **Perpetual inventory**: The products are transferred into an inventory account and are not expensed until used. Perpetual inventory is normally used in the warehouse and distribution departments. A perpetual system keeps track of current inventory figures. Many hospitals are moving toward perpetual inventory systems, which require diligent record keeping and precise inventory levels because of automated reordering processes.

Conducting Physical Inventory

Physical inventories account for all available supplies within a hospital. Many external companies provide inventory services that cannot only account for items, but provide location details within a line-item summary. Though effective, use of these companies can also be expensive. As such, many managers may be needed to conduct internal inventories within their hospitals. A process for internal inventories can be found in Chapter 6. Physical inventories can establish baseline valuations based on supplies on shelves. The process includes a thorough review of items on every shelf within a hospital, accounting for usable items, expired items, and items that require replacements. Once all items are accounted for, materials management staff will apply monetary values to inventory by matching products to current market prices, as well as the total value of items in house. Outcomes of physical inventory should be as follows:

- Identify reduction opportunities
- Identify items in inventory, but not accounted for in an item master
- Identify slow-moving or obsolete items, resulting in reduced future stock (reduced PAR levels)
- Identify excess items for removal
- Identify items without par location in MMIS

Use of handheld technology when conducting a physical inventory can create efficiencies and accuracy. Most hospitals use handheld computers that scan product barcodes, requiring staff to merely add volume numbers to scanned products. The information is then entered into a central computer that reorders supplies.

Managing your department's inventory will enable you to reduce overspending and more efficiently manage your materials. Be sure you understand the difference between expense upon receipt and perpetual inventory. Continually monitor your physical inventory to make sure items are accounted for and used effectively.

Supply Chain Metrics/Definitions

Commonly used supply chain metrics include:

- Supply availability is a percentage of purchase order lines delivered on time and in full quantities ordered to the closest point of use to the patient.
- Supply chain cost as a percentage of operating expense is a metric used to benchmark hospitals against similar facilities to see how well they are

operating. This figure incorporates facility size, type of facility, case mix level, and acuity. Supply chain cost calculates all supply chain expenses, including purchased services, medical surgical, medical device, pharmaceutical spending, and supply chain expenses as a percentage of total operating costs.

▓ Span of control is the total dollar amount of supply chain products and services under supply chain management, and total dollars spent on nonlabor supplies and services.

▓ Spend under contract is the percent of supply chain spend that is covered by a negotiated contract. Ninety-five percent of all regularly used products should be contract-based.

▓ Contract compliance is the percent of purchase order lines (PO lines) that can be associated with a specific contract. A real issue with rising supply costs ties back to when staff order products that are not on contract. These can include items that the vendor brings in.

▓ Contract adherence cycle time is the average number of days from the effective date of a contract, up until the point in which 80% of the funds spent is under the current contract.

▓ Supply chain operations costs are calculated as all fixed and variable costs as a percent of total expenditures, including contracting, transportation and logistics, warehouse and storeroom inventory holding costs, customer service, supplies, and purchase orders.

Understanding Purchase Orders

A PO is a document sent to a supplier or vendor authorizing shipment of a product to the customer at a specified price. As previously explained, POs are legally binding and should be used whenever ordering supplies because they provide pricing and volume information to use against received quantities.

The typical sections of a PO are as follows:

▓ Date

▓ PO number

▓ Names and addresses of both customer and the supplier/vendor

▓ Description of the items ordered, including costs and quantity

One final component of the PO process relates to capital purchases. Individual items not typically held to capital purchasing rules may be subjected to these statutes if requested quantities exceed capital spending caps. As such, it is important to keep total purchase order prices under consideration to avoid unnecessary capital purchase limitations.

SUMMARY

Nonlabor spending represents a large portion of departmental budgets and is a hospital's second-highest expense after labor. In today's economic environment, it is critical that department managers understand and participate in the oversight of supply and service costs as well as capital expenses. A clear understanding of the four links of a supply chain will allow departments to work together, improving the organization as a whole. Improving the function and participation of a VAT will further aid supply chain efficiencies. A broad understanding of management and inventory is essential for managing a department that provides quality patient care while staying within budget. Awareness of GPO agreements and working with physicians and clinicians toward optimizing the value of GPO relationships only adds to potential savings.

PART TWO

Conclusion

Nancy Bateman and Marilyn Connell

CASE STUDY: PHYSICIAN BUY-IN

Surgeons and other physicians are important participants in vendor standardization. This case study examines the reduction of vendors supplying total joint replacement supplies.

Orthopedics is an example of a complex service because surgeons build strong and lasting relationships with vendors. This often results in a surgeon's reluctance to change vendors because they become comfortable using the same vendors and implants regardless of patient needs. Many total-joint-implant vendors, however, offer comparable demand levels that provide similar outcomes. When beginning cost-saving initiatives it is imperative to use data to determine current vendor rates and usage.

A review of implant models will help to determine if the appropriate level of implant is selected according to the patient's age, health, and activity levels. High-end implants, which can cost more than double a medium- or low-level implant, should be used only when a patient is younger and requires long-term and highly active results. Older patients, who need the implant for palliative care, only need low-level demand implants for stability. In addition to the cost of prostheses and related components, hospitals should also consider the costs of cement, instrumentation, operating room time, length of the patient's hospitalization, nursing and rehabilitation, and other hospitalization costs.

With this information, surgeons receive a complete assessment of appropriate options and are more inclined to support low-cost options when applicable. Surgeons who do not agree to evaluate comparable implant vendors should be assessed on their contributions and overall performance measures, comparing this information to that of their peers. Hospital executives should demonstrate a surgeon's costs versus outcomes, highlighting any significant variances against targeted cost and quality levels. Surgeons may not be aware of their financial impact and may become more willing to support hospital efforts. Figures II.1 through II.4 display pricing and outcomes data, and were used in meetings with orthopedic surgeons at the hospital. Service-line analysis was performed as a baseline for costs and outcomes against regional and national best practices. Understanding what vendors currently use, and the costs associated with these vendors, established that price reductions would result in an annual savings of $1.5 million.

Figures II.1 through II.4 were used to convince physicians to partner with their hospitals toward mutual improvements in cost and quality outcomes.

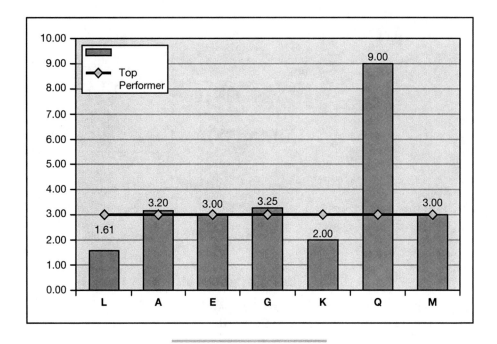

FIGURE II.1
ALOS by Physician—Hips

Figure II.1 compared surgeons in relation to the patient length of stay for their total hip cases. Figures II.2 and II.3 show current vendor pricing for implants compared to the total hospital reimbursement for patient care. In order not to lose money, the cost of the implants should not be greater than 35% to 38% of the total reimbursement.

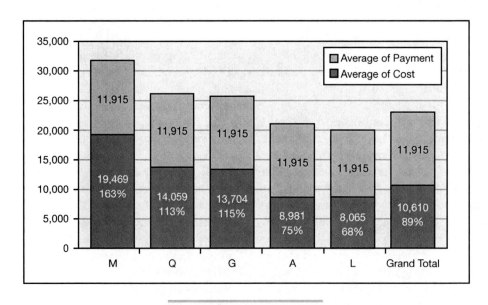

FIGURE II.2
Community Total Hip Implant Costs as a Percent of Medicare Reimbursement

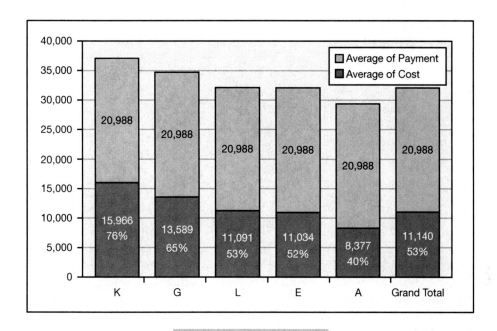

FIGURE II.3
Community Total Hip Implant Costs as a Percent of Commercial Reimbursement

Figure II.4 demonstrates implant costs per surgeon compared with top quartile pricing for the same implants and vendors. In all but one case, surgeon implant costs are higher than market pricing in their local, regional, and national areas.

A total of 12 surgeons were performing total joint replacements within this community hospital, and all but two were willing to evaluate new vendors should

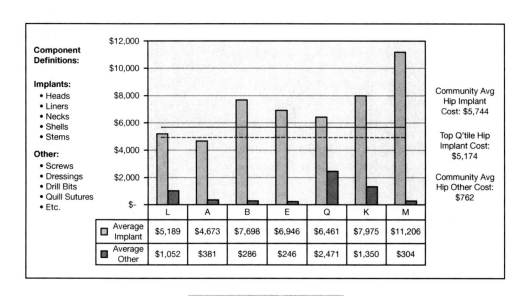

FIGURE II.4
Average Hip Implant Expense by Physician

their current vendor refuse to meet market-identified pricing. Surgeons were then provided with two options: reduce or substitute vendors or open the vendor field to three and negotiate a price cap in advance with each. Surgeons opted to pursue the capped model because the achieved savings would allow the hospital to purchase new technologies and choose from a larger product mix. The hospital saved $1.8 million through a combination of reduced implant costs and ancillary supplies. Improvements in surgery usage and preassessment processes allowed for improved quality outcomes for patients.

CONCLUSION

To effectively acquire new supplies, services, and capital equipment, the Nurse Manager must understand the supply chain and know where money is being spent. Consistent vigilance of wasted materials and avoiding that waste will diminish unnecessary budget drain. Nurse Managers must manage the budget, with the support of the value analysis team and group purchasing organizations, to deliver the best possible price for quality products and help keep budget expenditures in check. Other important management skills that help to effectively manage your budget include becoming familiar with various contracts and methods for working with vendors; being aware of physician and clinician involvement to promote optimal communication; and keeping accurate inventory records and routinely adjusting PAR levels to reflect actual needs to stay within budget.

PART THREE

Finance

Nancy Bateman and Pam Wright

Understanding health care finance is essential to creating and maintaining a productive budget. Thus, this part introduces the finance department and its operations. Content includes communication strategies, accounting concepts, financial statements, and budgeting processes, with monthly and annual variance analyses. Creating annual budgets is not only a good management tool but it also helps to determine and report any variances. Purchasing, in coordination with the finance department, enables you to get the best product at the best price. Understanding the financial side of purchasing also helps when reimbursements are necessary. Chapter 7 introduces the reader to the world of reimbursement for an understanding of how we are paid for the care we deliver. Finally, managed care is an integral part in controlling medical costs by allowing only medically necessary services to be provided in the most cost-effective setting.

Whether the reader is a professional budgeter or just starting out, Part III of this book introduces the basics and then builds to the more sophisticated budgeting concepts.

6

Annual Budgeting and Purchasing as Part of Health Care Finance

Nancy Bateman and Pam Wright

Depending on the size of a facility, a finance department may be comprised of 3 to 50 employees. The chief financial officer (CFO) is the head of the department and typically reports to the company president. Other finance department employees may include a controller, several financial analysts, and many staff accountants. The primary responsibility of the CFO and the finance department is to safeguard the assets of the company by maintaining the company's financial records. The finance department prepares financial statements that detail the historical results of the company's operations, and budgets that detail anticipated results. These financial reports provide information used in decision-making processes.

LEARNING OBJECTIVES

1. Gain an understanding of the finance department and its role in hospital operations.
2. Become familiar with financial reporting.
3. Prepare department budgets using the different financial reports provided by your finance department.
4. Recognize your role in the budget process.
5. Identify and report budget versus actual variances.
6. Define a purchase order (PO) and identify the information needed to complete it.
7. Understand the ordering process from the perspective of the finance department.
8. Describe the relationship between finance's needs and inventory.

UNDERSTANDING HEALTH CARE FINANCE

Financial Statements

There are three primary financial statements: balance sheets, income statements, and statements of cash flow. These statements may be prepared for the company as a whole or on an individual departmental basis.

Balance Sheets

The balance sheet is a snapshot of a company's assets, liabilities, and equity at a specific point in time. Assets are items owned by the company such as cash, accounts receivable, and inventory. Liabilities represent money that a company owes to others, including accounts payable and notes payable. Equity is the difference between total assets and total liabilities. Table 6.1 is an example of a consolidated balance sheet. In this example, the balance sheet is consolidated because the system has more than one facility. Summarizing all of the results, Table 6.1 provides a snapshot of what is happening across the entire system at once.

Income (Profit and Loss) Statements

An income statement—also referred to as a profit and loss (P&L) statement—details the results of the company's operations during a specific period. These periods vary, usually covering a month, a quarter, or a year. The income statement shows the company's revenues, expenses, and net income or loss. Income statements are typically prepared for each department on a monthly basis and are compared to budgeted amounts, listing each expense compared to the total spending to date against what was budgeted or expected to be spent. The financial difference is considered the variance, hence the reason this statement can also be referred to as a *variance report.* Table 6.2 is an example showing the variances for the month of August and year to date (YTD) against the same period for the previous year and month.

Statement of Cash Flows

The *statement of cash flows* summarizes the company's amount of cash on hand to pay bills for a period that is consistent with the income statement. Specifically, this statement shows the primary sources and uses of company funds.

The finance department uses information from the general ledger (GL) to prepare financial statements. A GL is a collection of individual accounts that supports the value of the items shown in the financial statements. A company may have anywhere from 25 to 1,000 accounts within its GL. Typically, there are specific accounts for assets, liabilities, revenues, and expenses. Transactions reflecting operational activities are detailed within each account. For example, a utility expense account would include all expenses associated with the company's electric bills.

Common Finance Terms

A list of common finance terms found within a hospital's financial operations could include the following:

- **Generally accepted accounting principles (GAAP)**—A set of rules, standards, and procedures dictating the proper way to prepare financial statements and related disclosures. This is not typically a concern for nonfinance employees.

TABLE 6.1
Consolidated Balance Statement

											244	Days to date
			CONSOLIDATED BALANCE SHEET									
			As of August 31, 2009									
					Urgent	Specialty					Current	PY
	Site A	Site B	Site C	Cares	Clinics	Site D	Site E	Foundation	Elim.		Total	Total
ASSETS												
Current Assets:												
Cash and Investments	(11,723,424)	22,566,369	1,862,016	6,053	18,568	1,962	139,631	(381,510)	-		12,489,665	24,305,619
Accounts Receivable - Net	-	27,995,541	7,041,031	364,848	509,375	262	6,410	-	-		35,917,467	35,735,023
Third Party Settlement Receivables	-	829,354	125,696	-	-	-	-	-	-		955,050	2,138,109
Inventories	562,515	5,769,567	1,077,989	-	-	-	-	-	-		7,410,071	7,521,068
Prepaids	1,100,412	1,905,948	412,968	10,753	15,086	-	12,333	337	-		3,457,837	2,661,931
Funds Held by Trustee	479,317	3,580,657	2,938,448	-	-	-	-	-	-		6,998,422	9,684,418
Receivables from Affiliates	29,285,158	66,974	11	-	-	2,473	100,000	-	(29,454,615)		1	-
Other Current Assets and Receivables	2,293,427	821,667	3,444,500	1,049	271	523	-	-	-		6,558,437	2,343,413
Current Portion of Non Current Assets	98,012	106,038	-	-	-	-	-	-	-		204,080	145,176
Total Current Assets	22,092,447	63,642,115	16,902,659	382,703	543,300	5,220	258,374	(381,173)	(29,454,615)		73,991,030	84,534,757
Board Designated Assets:												
Cash and Investments	583,540	3,193,554	370,859	-	-	-	-	-	-		4,147,953	4,756,480
Funds Held by Trustee	567,317	7,000,208	6,823,960	-	-	-	-	-	-		14,391,485	7,432,282
Total Board Designated Assets	1,150,857	10,193,762	7,194,819	-	-	-	-	-	-		18,539,438	12,188,762
Property, Plant & Equipment:												
Property, Plant and Equipment	14,808,070	228,026,256	71,345,870	655,835	118,508	33,230	88,620	-	-		315,076,389	302,138,501
Accumulated Depreciation	(11,637,677)	(140,828,900)	(36,396,826)	(335,963)	(75,050)	(33,230)	(38,452)	-	-		(189,346,098)	(178,037,198)
Net Property, Plant and Equipment	3,170,393	87,197,356	34,949,044	319,872	43,458	-	50,168	-	-		125,730,291	124,101,303
Other Assets:												
Cash, Investments, and Reserves	175,834	2,789,853	111,841	-	-	17,394	-	7,011,412	-		10,106,334	11,409,581
Notes Receivable, net	4,429,930	1,196,997	9,127	-	-	-	-	-	-		5,636,054	7,246,192
Investments in Joint Ventures	1,420,918	5,534,330	368,381	-	-	-	-	-	-		7,323,629	9,239,085
Unamortized Financing Costs	81,350	580,358	86,468	-	-	-	-	-	-		748,176	907,264
Investments in Subsidiary	1,326,038	-	-	-	-	103,326	-	-	(1,429,364)		-	-
Other Assets	-	-	-	-	-	-	-	-	-		-	-
Total Other Assets	7,434,070	10,101,538	575,817	-	-	120,720	-	7,011,412	(1,429,364)		23,814,193	28,802,122
Total Assets	33,847,767	171,134,771	59,622,339	702,575	586,758	125,940	308,542	6,630,239	(30,883,979)		242,074,952	249,626,944
											48,133,859	57,588,380
Key Statistical Indicators:	Description:									Targets		
Days cash on hand	Operating cash & investment / Total operating expenses less: bad debt, depreciation & interest									90.0	27.6	49.7
Days revenue in accounts receivable	Net accounts receivable / Net patient service revenues less bad debts									60.0	56.6	58.0
Cushion ratio	Cash & investments plus funds held by trustee / Total annual debt service										2.6	3.1
Cash to debt (%)	Cash & investments plus funds held by trustee / Total LT debt outstanding less current maturities										31%	49%
Days supplies in inventory	Inventory / Supplies expense										50.5	51.5
LIABILITIES												
Current Liabilities:												
Accounts Payable	1,334,757	4,580,270	477,203	7,394	25,952	-	4,391	284,190	-		6,714,157	8,463,299
Payroll and Payroll Related Liabilities	15,071,144	1,389,420	465,013	7,562	135,545	-	22,468	-	-		16,991,152	15,456,855
Third Party Settlement Payables	-	365,663	26,803	-	-	-	-	-	-		392,468	596,968
Affiliate Payables	100,000	-	24,765,886	1,008,253	3,126,116	219,642	234,718	-	(29,454,615)		-	-
Interest and Other Payables	487,749	994,070	189,908	5,197	2,773	-	1,451	-	-		1,681,148	31,262,169
Curr Portion of Long Term Liabilities	498,991	5,514,584	3,343,274	-	-	-	-	-	-		9,356,849	7,577,621
Total Current Liabilities	17,492,641	12,544,009	29,268,087	1,028,406	3,290,386	219,642	263,028	284,190	(29,454,615)		34,935,774	63,356,912
Long-Term Liabilities:												
Bonds/Capital Lease Obligations	6,937,349	64,978,454	33,153,261	-	-	-	-	-	-		105,069,064	64,720,003
Other LT liabilities	3,884,947	4,935,373	2,926,178	-	-	-	-	303,777	-		12,050,275	19,089,394
Less: Curr Portion of LT Liabilities	(498,991)	(5,514,584)	(3,343,275)	-	-	-	-	-	-		(9,356,850)	(7,577,622)
Net Long Term Debt	10,323,305	64,399,243	32,736,164	-	-	-	-	303,777	-		107,762,489	76,231,773
Fund Balance and Retained Earnings	6,031,821	94,191,519	(2,381,912)	(325,831)	(2,703,628)	(93,702)	45,514	6,042,272	(1,429,364)		99,376,689	110,038,259
Total Liabilities and Fund Balance	33,847,767	171,134,771	59,622,339	702,575	586,758	125,940	308,542	6,630,239	(30,883,979)		242,074,952	249,626,944

TABLE 6.2
Variance Report

		August 04'	August 03'			YTD August 04'	Prior YTD	
Revenue:		Actual	Actual	% Var		Actual	Actual	% Var
Inpatient Revenue		25,189,289	20,075,709	25.5%		183,942,779	177,690,382	3.5%
Outpatient Revenue		16,209,048	13,255,446	22.3%		105,992,841	107,733,709	-1.6%
Total Patient Revenue (Charges)		41,398,337	33,331,155	24.2%		289,935,620	285,424,091	1.6%
Less: Deductions from Revenue		(22,208,793)	(14,415,837)	54.1%		(135,209,339)	(135,140,424)	0.1%
Net Patient Revenue		19,189,544	18,915,318	1.5%		154,726,281	150,283,667	3.0%
Other Operating Revenue		351,897	514,233	-31.6%		3,606,090	4,964,534	-27.4%
Total Net Revenue		19,541,441	19,429,551	0.6%		158,332,371	155,248,201	2.0%
Operating Expenses:								
Salaries		6,854,315	7,335,073	-6.6%		61,545,220	62,635,615	-1.7%
Employee Benefits		1,727,611	1,921,274	-10.1%		12,512,008	13,532,119	-7.5%
Total Salaries and Benefits		8,581,926	9,256,347	-7.3%		74,057,228	76,167,734	-2.8%
Professional Fees		1,943,917	570,687	240.6%		10,190,810	4,513,066	125.8%
- elimination of OI related fees		(924,193)	-			(3,535,351)	-	
Supplies		4,432,365	4,016,824	10.4%		35,808,957	35,628,924	0.5%
Utilities		62,124	56,472	10.0%		438,568	1,284,977	-65.9%
Purchased Services-Outside		1,960,255	1,785,695	9.8%		15,119,980	11,992,113	26.1%
Purchased Services-Other		455,119	414,756	9.7%		3,442,795	3,282,896	4.9%
Provision for Bad Debts		2,162,449	521,691	314.5%		10,902,269	5,189,551	110.1%
Depreciation		1,377,906	1,008,100	36.7%		10,790,683	8,876,512	21.6%
Rental and Leases		242,112	141,111	71.6%		2,022,932	1,489,403	35.8%
Insurance		288,606	401,153	-28.1%		2,604,817	1,957,100	33.1%
Interest Expense		422,481	375,875	12.4%		3,512,438	2,882,754	21.8%
Other Direct Expense		345,510	277,176	24.7%		3,078,140	3,311,620	-7.1%
(Gain/Loss on Medstar)		35,271	-			234,072	(265,076)	
Total Operating Expenses		21,385,848	18,825,887	13.6%		168,668,338	156,311,574	7.9%
Gain (Loss) from Operations		(1,844,407)	603,664	-405.5%		(10,335,967)	(1,063,373)	872.0%
Non-Operating/Other Gains (Losses)								
Interest/Dividends/Contributions		43,990	45,731	-3.8%		853,164	544,127	56.8%
INHS/Joint Ventures/Other Gain/(Loss)		(175,909)	(105,963)	66.0%		(682,705)	579,657	
Unrealized G/L on Investments		(67,420)	(29,111)			(3,372)	153,208	
Prior Period/Extraordinary/OI related		(924,193)	-			(1,506,609)	4,491,747	
Total Other Gains/Losses		(1,123,532)	(89,343)			(1,339,522)	5,768,739	
Net Gain (Loss)		(2,967,939)	514,321			(11,675,489)	4,705,366	
Operating Margin - %		-9.61%	3.19%			-6.68%	-0.71%	
Average Daily Census		197.3	211.5	-6.7%		216.2	230.1	-6.0%
	Chrg. Adj.				Chrg. Adj.			
Adjusted Patient Days (APD)	9,501	10,217	10,648	-4.1%	80,911	81,627	87,938	-7.2%
Net Revenue/APD	$ 1,792	$ 1,667	$ 1,727	-3.5%	$ 1,778	$ 1,762	$ 1,650	6.8%
Salaries & Benefits/APD	$ 903	$ 840	$ 869	-3.4%	$ 915	$ 907	$ 866	4.8%
Supplies/APD	$ 467	$ 434	$ 377	15.0%	$ 443	$ 439	$ 405	8.3%

▣ **Return on investment (ROI)**—Most often reported as a percentage, it is the revenue earned as divided by the amount invested for a project or capital purchase.

▣ **Inventory**—A detailed list of types and costs of materials on hand. In health care, this may be the total of all tangible goods and property. The inventory value must be counted and reported at the end of each accounting period. The nonlabor chapter discussed inventory as a measure of all supplies purchased and held until use. The value of inventory is determined by the valuation method within a facility. Typically, inventory will be stated at the lowest cost or market value, ensuring that inventory values are not overstated. Because inventory is often the largest asset on hospital balance sheets, its value is tracked on a daily basis. Daily inventory tracking is referred to as "perpetual inventory," and is also explained in the preceding chapter. The implementation of perpetual inventory systems is highly recommended within health care because of the inability to forecast materials usage. Further information on inventories can be found in Chapter 5.

▣ **Prepaids**—Short for prepaid expenses. Prepaids refers to payments made in advance for items such as rent, insurance premiums, and interest. Prepaids are included as assets on balance sheets. They will be amortized (i.e., written off) to expenses as their related obligations become current.

▣ **Amortization**—The process of writing off the cost of an asset's useful life. Prepaid expenses are typically amortized over a period of 1 to 3 months. Intangible assets—defined next—are amortized over a period of 1 to 15 years.

▣ **Intangible asset**—Refers to nonphysical items (i.e., intellectual property, patents, or trademarks). The value of an intangible asset is determined initially by contracts or other agreements. Intangible assets are reviewed annually to ensure that their value is both reasonable and realizable to the hospital.

▣ **Depreciation**—Represents the process of writing off the costs of tangible assets over their useful lives. Depreciation is not to be confused with amortization, which deals primarily with intangible assets. Tangible assets are buildings, equipment, or anything that has a long-term physical existence and is required for the business to operate, but is not sold to customers. Useful lives of these assets range from 3 to 30 years. These assets are usually seen in balance sheets as plant operations or capital equipment. Tangible assets can be used to secure loans versus intangible assets that cannot be used as collateral.

▣ **Notes receivable (NR)**—These represent amounts due from third parties, and are typically documented via written agreements or contracts. Notes receivable will be classified as current assets if the funds are expected to be collected within the next 12 months and as noncurrent if the collection period is anticipated to be greater than 1 year.

▣ **Days in accounts receivable (AR)**—The number of days it takes for a facility to process and collect payments. AR is calculated by dividing sales by average accounts receivable. A high number in this line item indicates that the hospital may have collection issues with its customers.

▣ **Cushion ratio**—This is the balance of net cash flow after all debt has been paid.

- **Operating margin**—Noted again as a percentage, this is gross margin (revenue minus costs to operate) after subtracting depreciation and taxes.

- **Profit margin**—A percentage reflecting the profitability of an organization after taxes and operating costs.

- **Revenue growth**—Another percentage tracked to reflect organizational performance. This metric compares the revenue from the current reporting period to that of the last reporting period. Revenue growth is calculated using current revenues subtracted by the previous period's revenue and then divided by the previous period's revenue.

- **Net cash flow**—Net cash flow is the change between a current ending cash balance and the cash balance at the end of the last reporting period. Net cash flow is tracked either monthly or by reporting period.

- **Adjusted patient days (APD)**—Used to monitor statistics and calculate unit-of-service metrics. Patient days are the number of patients cared for in a 24-hour period. APD takes this calculation a step further and incorporates care for outpatients, ensuring that gross revenue is accurately reflected. The formula to determine APD is in patient days multiplied by gross patient revenue, with that total divided by inpatient revenue.

- **Cost center (CC)**—The department code or geographically defined area where all direct and indirect costs are allocated. Department managers will be assigned cost center codes and will list all expenses according to predetermined codes.

- **Subaccount**—Subaccounts help separate expenses within a cost center. Maintaining separate subaccounts allow managers to track specific spending trends, helping them locate budget variances and overages.

- **Direct costs**—Expenses that are directly attributed specific cost centers such as labor or supplies.

- **Indirect costs**—Expenses that are difficult to assign to a single cost center are typically those which are shared by several departments. Indirect costs would include facility costs for an entire hospital, such as advertising or maintenance.

- **Variable costs**—These are expenses that change based on department activity. Variable costs include utilities and supplies (high census would require more supplies and summer versus winter affects utility usage).

- **Fixed costs**—Refers to expenses that may vary over time, but do not change from an accounting perspective.

Understanding the health care side of finance will help you create a budget that makes quality purchases that result in profit to your department. Know how to read your financial income (profit and loss [P&L]) statements, and your system of cash flows. Being comfortable with the common finance terms will also be beneficial when negotiating contracts.

Strategic Planning

In addition to common finance vocabulary, strategic planning and operating budgets support the direction of an organization's budget and overall growth. The purpose of strategic planning is to set company goals for current and future periods focusing on needs, risks, and company opportunities. Strategic planning identifies key decisions for administrators, establishing guidelines and deadlines for accomplishing goals. The strategic plan is a blueprint used by a company's management to keep it on the right course to achieving objectives.

Operating Budgets

The operating budget is a key component to a company's strategic plan, defining the company's performance and operational objectives. Budgets are typically prepared on an annual basis and include balance sheets, income statements, and statements of cash flows for each department and for the company as a whole. Operating budgets include monthly, quarterly, and year-to-date data. This discussion will focus on departmental income statements because they are a likely area of responsibility. Table 6.3 provides an example of an annual budget for one department. In Table 6.3, expenses have been separated by category and month. This enables future detailed analysis of budgeted values versus actual results.

CREATING ANNUAL BUDGETS

Preparing a complete departmental budget may seem tedious and overly detail-oriented, but it is essential for the overall viability of an organization.

Budgets are typically prepared by finance departments, with significant input from each operating department. Depending on the organization, responsibilities may range from providing commentary on existing budgets to preparing initial drafts of future departmental budgets.

Review of Prior-Period Operating Results

The first step in the budgeting process is a review of prior-period operating results. It is important to pay close attention to operating trends and variances between periods because it will be necessary to determine their causes, and take these factors into consideration when setting future budget amounts. Next, consider departmental business activities for the next year: Will the department be expanding its personnel or activities? Will new products or services be introduced? Conversely, will the department's operations be reduced because of a reduction in workforce or a phasing out of services?

Once the scope of a department's operations is determined, it is time to address the timing of these activities. Certain costs are recurring and similar in amount, although other costs are seasonal, biyearly, or yearly.

Taking all of these factors into consideration, managers should map out each expense category on a monthly basis, comparing totals in each category to those from prior periods while ensuring that variances can be explained. Also, consider whether a budget, as proposed, fits within a company's direction for the upcoming year. If the company officers have communicated that they will implement expense reductions across the board, a budget should reflect this.

Completed budgets are then submitted to finance departments for review. The finance department combines departmental budgets and decides whether the

TABLE 6.3
Annual Department Budget

Tatum Hospital
Department A
Operation Plan
For the Year Ended 12/31/11

	Jan	Feb	Mar	Apr	May	Jun	Jul	Aug	Sep	Oct	Nov	Dec	FY 2011
Salaries	12,000	12,000	12,000	12,000	12,000	12,000	15,000	15,000	15,000	15,000	15,000	15,000	162,000
Employee benefits	2,000	2,000	2,000	2,000	2,000	2,000	3,000	3,000	3,000	3,000	3,000	3,000	30,000
Office supplies	2,500	2,500	2,500	2,500	2,500	2,500	2,500	2,500	2,500	2,500	2,500	2,500	30,000
Consulting expense	1,500	–	1,500	–	1,500	–	1,500	1,500	1,500	1,500	1,500	1,500	13,500
Marketing expense	–	–	2,000	–	–	2,500	3,000	–	–	5,000	–	–	12,000
Travel	500	500	500	500	500	500	500	500	500	500	500	500	6,000
Shipping expense	1,000	1,000	1,000	1,000	1,000	1,000	1,000	1,000	1,000	1,000	1,000	1,000	12,000
Total	19,500	18,000	21,500	18,000	19,500	20,500	26,500	23,500	23,500	28,500	23,500	23,500	266,000

company's strategic objectives are being addressed appropriately, and whether the proposed activity levels of each department are consistent. This process may take one to two weeks, depending on the size of the hospital. On completion of budget reviews, the finance department returns budgets to department heads, usually including modifications. These changes do not reflect the quality of a budget, but rather the incorporation of new data that might not have been included during the first pass. Managers are then able to discuss modifications with the finance department.

Budget Versus Actual Analysis

Managers are responsible for reporting their department's actual results versus budgeted performance on a monthly basis. Typically, the finance department will provide a report similar to that found in Table 6.4, which demonstrates the results of a monthly budget against actual spending.

Managers are responsible for explaining significant budget variances. For example, actual salary expenses may be higher than budgeted expenses because of additional hires after the completion of the budget. It is often helpful to notify the finance department of significant budget variances as they arise.

Though managing both operational and financial aspects of a department can be a daunting task, an understanding of the basics can lead to successful financial reporting and budgeting processes. If possible, find a finance department employee who can provide guidance and support as a relationship is established. This contact may also become a departmental advocate on budgeting issues.

When creating an annual budget, make sure you are constantly analyzing budget versus actual spent. It may seem like a tedious task, but determining and reporting variances will allow you to assess the goals, needs, and risks that may affect your department. A well-organized and thought-out annual budget will result in a surplus allowing for more advanced financial opportunities in the future.

TABLE 6.4
Budget Versus Actual Report

Tatum Hospital
Department A
Operating Results
For the Month Ended January 31, 2011

	Budget	Actual	Variance
Salaries	12,000	15,000	(3,000)
Employee benefits	2,000	3,500	(1,500)
Office supplies	2,500	2,000	500
Consulting expense	1,500	1,200	300
Marketing expense	–	4,000	(4,000)
Travel	500	200	300
Shipping expense	1,000	222	778
Total	19,500	26,122	(6,622)

PURCHASING CONSIDERATIONS FROM THE FINANCE SIDE

To effectively manage a department, medical and office supplies must be physically available when necessary, but must not be stored in excessive quantities. A hospital's purchasing department (part of materials management) will help with this balancing act. The purchasing department monitors suppliers and procures materials at competitive prices.

Although the purchasing department processes the orders, they must conform to the requirements set forth by the finance department. Such a purchase of materials typically calls for the creation of a purchase order (PO). As illustrated in Figure 6.1, a PO includes all information pertinent to a department's need for a product. Most facilities have a standard PO form that can be filled in, and all order forms require some kind of approval before processing. Different management levels have increasing levels of approval, advanced levels of approval are required for increasingly expensive items. A PO approval structure may look like the following:

Department head	$500
Division head	$5,000
Vice president	$25,000
President	$100,000

A purchasing department can provide a list of vendors and product numbers. Certain facilities will require a department to complete PO forms, while others simply request department leaders to pass along information to the purchasing department, who will then complete the appropriate documentation.

The Ordering Process

Purchasing departments maintain approved supplier lists including all vendors who have demonstrated their ability to meet a hospital's specified quality requirements. Typically, orders are only placed with suppliers on this list, although new vendors may be added to the approved supplier list after meeting the criteria specified by the department.

The purchasing department is responsible for procuring reasonable quantities of materials at the lowest prices available. Prior to the initial order of a new product, the purchasing department will obtain bids from several vendors, which will include product quantities, pricing, delivery timing, and payment terms. Each bid is then evaluated and a determination is made regarding which vendor offers the best combination of terms. Once this determination is made, the facility will execute a purchase contract with the vendor for a specified time and quantity.

Based on existing sales contracts, a purchasing department will notify a requestor of the product quantities and delivery schedules for the requested materials. It is important to track product usage against these schedules to prevent shortages or buildups. If a department is at risk for either of these scenarios, it is necessary to contact the purchasing department to manage the situation.

Many facilities require monthly or quarterly physical inventories to maintain additional control over departmental supplies and materials. For a thorough explanation of inventory processes, refer to the preceding chapter's segment on inventory management. Part and parcel to the process are inventory forms as demonstrated in Table 6.5.

XXX Hospital				PURCHASE ORDER	
			DATE:	3/31/2011	
			P.O. #	[123456]	

[Stress Address]
[City, ST ZIP]
Phone: [000-000-0000]
Fax: [000-000-0000]

VENDOR	SHIP TO
ABC Company	Sue Purchaser
Hospital Supplies Division	XXX Hospital
2245 Supply Avenue	555 Hospital Circle
Phoenix, AZ 85008	Phoenix, AZ 85001
(480) 222-3333	(602) 555-2222

REQUISTIONER	SHIP VIA	F.O.B.	SHIPPING TERMS

ITEM #	DESCRIPTION	QTY	UNIT PRICE	TOTAL
[23423423]	Product XYZ	15	150.00	2,250.00
[45645645]	Product ABC	1	75.00	75.00
				–
				–
				–
				–
				–
				–
				–
				–
				–
				–

Other Comments or Special Instructions

SUBTOTAL	$	2,325.00
TAX RATE		6.875%
TAX	$	159.84
S & H	$	250.00
OTHER	$	–
TOTAL	$	2,734.84

Authorized by   Date

If you have any questions about this purchase order, please contact

FIGURE 6.1
Sample Purchase Order Form

TABLE 6.5
Inventory Form

ABC Hospital
Department X
January 31, 20xx

Part Number	Description	Quantity
223	Product A	
435	Product B	
707	Product C	
760	Product D	
828	Product E	
127	Product F	
406	Product G	
168	Product H	

Completed By _____

Title _____

Typically, completed physical inventory forms are submitted to the finance department for review and analysis, but keeping track of physical inventory can help managers track their own monthly or quarterly inventory levels as demonstrated in Table 6.6.

Trends in inventory levels can provide valuable information related to a department. For example, in Table 6.6, it appears that the quantity on hand of Product H

TABLE 6.6
Physical Inventory Form

ABC Hospital
Department X

Part Number	Description	Quantity on Hand			
		March 20xx	June 20xx	Sept 20xx	Dec 20xx
223	Product A	15	18	25	20
435	Product B	66	22	66	20
707	Product C	23	23	23	24
760	Product D	10	1	5	20
828	Product E	55	75	100	125
127	Product F	55	22	11	1
406	Product G	200	300	250	200
168	Product H	250	250	330	350

is growing. This indicates that the quantities of this product ordered should be reduced, but more importantly, that this accumulation of inventory may indicate a declining demand for the service associated with the product. Conversely, the quantity on hand of Product F has declined significantly. This signals a future potential shortage of this product. This decline in quantity could be the result of a department phasing out the use of the product, or it could be an indication of a problem with the vendor. In any event, both trends require follow-up analysis and should be brought to the attention of both materials management and purchasing departments.

SUMMARY

Understanding purchasing from the financial side requires that you have a thorough understanding of POs including how to request and process them. Coordinating the ordering process with monthly or quarterly physical inventories allows you to identify trends that may become opportunities for saving money on supplies. To acquire the newest technologies at the best prices it is imperative that you are able to communicate with the finance department.

7

Patient Care Reimbursement

Nancy Bateman and Anna Raneses

An important component of the business of nursing is understanding reimbursement for patient care. Most commercial payers base their reimbursement off of the government prospective payment system. This chapter will review the evolution of the prospective payment system and its structure. Although the details around the payment structure may seem dry and confusing, it is important to gain as much knowledge as possible about them, specifically regarding patient stays and resource consumption. With government payment systems, reimbursement is designed to cover all hospital care. The ability to understand what is covered and the documentation required to assign correct labels to each patient will positively or negatively affect your overall budget. Knowing the difference between governmental and commercial insurance also will help ensure that coding adheres to the diagnosis-related group (DRG) payment system structure when reporting elements that concern diagnosis and procedures. Familiarity with reimbursement methods, managed care contracts, and basic contract terminology will facilitate your ability to improve your departments' efficiency.

LEARNING OBJECTIVES

1. Understanding the prospective payment system.
2. Define the role of diagnosis-related groups (DRGs) in health care reimbursement.
3. Understand case mix and how this ties to DRGs.
4. Define managed care and the negotiation process for managed care contracts.
5. Articulate the components of managed care contracts.
6. List the legal components of managed care contracts.

CENTERS FOR MEDICARE AND MEDICAID SERVICES REIMBURSEMENT

Medicare and Medicaid Reimbursements

The Centers for Medicare and Medicaid Services (CMS), originally known as Medicare and Medicaid, was established in 1965. Medicare insures adults older than the age of 65 and disabled individuals, whereas Medicaid provides insurance for all patients who are unable to afford commercial insurance.

CMS pays hospitals for inpatient stays according to the DRGs assigned to that patient based on their diagnosis. CMS makes changes to DRG classifications yearly, and health care reform legislation promises to make even more changes. Many of the examples within this chapter, when tied to a specific DRG, may not be applicable from one year to the next. For current information on DRG classifications or their associated rules and regulations, staff members should work with health information departments within their health care institution.

Uniform Hospital Discharge Data Sets

Before discussing the DRG payment system structure, an understanding of the Uniform Hospital Discharge Data Set (UHDDS) elements used in the system is necessary. UHDDS definitions are used by acute care hospitals to report inpatient data in a standardized manner. UHDDS data elements used in DRG classification are described below, including various diagnoses and related procedures. Proper DRG assignment and resulting reimbursement are dependent on reporting these elements correctly.

- Diagnoses: All diagnoses that affect the current hospital stay are to be reported. Principal diagnosis is defined as "that condition established after study to be chiefly responsible for occasioning the admission of the patient to the hospital for care."

- Other (additional) diagnoses are defined as "all conditions that coexist at the time of admission, that develop subsequently, or that affect the treatment received and/or the length of stay."

- Diagnoses related to an earlier episode of care, which have no bearing on the current hospital stay, are to be excluded. For reporting purposes, the definition for "other diagnoses" is interpreted as additional conditions that affect patient care in terms of requiring clinical evaluation, therapeutic treatment, diagnostic procedures, extended length of hospital stay, or increased nursing care and/or monitoring.

- Procedures: All significant procedures are to be reported. Significant procedures are those that are surgical in nature, carry a procedural risk, carry an anesthetic risk, or require specialized training. The principal procedure is one that was performed for definitive treatment rather than one performed for diagnostic or exploratory purposes, or was necessary to take care of a complication. If there appears to be two procedures that meet the above definition, then the one most related to the principal diagnosis should be selected as the principal procedure. Under Inpatient Prospective Payment System (IPPS) all procedures potentially affecting payment must be reported (HSS, 2006).

Inappropriately applied coding in the DRG payment system can mean reduced reimbursement to the hospital. The discussion that follows is provided with permission from the 3M Health Information Systems to avoid this situation. 3M offers software that supports coders in applying appropriate codes for reimbursement (Averill et al., 2003). This article on the history of DRGs was first published in 2003 and offers detailed background on the development and application of DRGs for reimbursement. Keep in mind this background is based off of the CMS Version 20, and as of 2010, we are up to Version 27. Fortunately, although DRG codes may change, the system has remained the same and remains our focus here.[1]

The Role of Diagnosis-Related Groups in Patient Care Reimbursement

The DRGs are a patient classification scheme that relates patient treatments to hospital costs. There are three major DRG versions currently in use: basic DRGs, All-Patient DRGs (AP-DRGs), and All-Patient Refined DRGs (APR-DRGs). The basic DRGs are used by the CMS for hospital payment to Medicare beneficiaries, AP-DRGs are an expansion of the basic DRGs to be more representative of the non-Medicare population, and APR-DRGs incorporate severity of illness subclasses into the AP-DRGs. Because the APR-DRGs include both the CMS DRGs and the AP-DRGs, the development of all three versions of the DRGs will be reviewed.

History

The design and development of the DRGs began in the late 1960s at Yale University to create an effective framework for monitoring the quality of care and the utilization of services in a hospital setting. The first large-scale application of DRGs occurred in New Jersey during the late 1970s as the basis of a prospective payment system (PPS), in which hospitals were reimbursed a fixed specific amount for each patient. In 1982, the Tax Equity and Fiscal Responsibility Act modified the Section 223 Medicare hospital reimbursement limits to include a case mix adjustment based on DRGs. In 1983, Congress amended the Social Security Act to include a national DRG-based hospital PPS for all Medicare patients.

The process of forming the original DRGs began by dividing all possible principal diagnoses into mutually exclusive principal diagnosis categories referred to as *major diagnostic categories* (MDCs). MDCs were formed by physician panels as the first step toward ensuring that the DRGs would be clinically coherent. The diagnoses in each MDC correspond to a single organ system or etiology and, in general, are associated with a particular medical specialty. Thus, in order to maintain the requirement of clinical coherence, no final DRG could contain patients in different MDCs. In general, each MDC was constructed to correspond to a major organ system (e.g., respiratory system, circulatory system, digestive system) rather than etiology (e.g., malignancies, infectious diseases). This approach was used because clinical care is generally organized in accordance with the organ system affected, rather than the etiology. Diseases involving both a particular organ system and a particular etiology (e.g., malignant neoplasm of the kidney) were assigned to the MDC corresponding to the organ system involved. However, not all diseases or disorders could be assigned to an organ system-based MDC and a number of residual MDCs were created. Once the medical and surgical groups for an MDC were formed, each patient group was evaluated to determine if complications, comorbidities, or the patient's age would consistently affect the consumption of hospital resources. Physician panels classified each diagnosis code based on whether the diagnosis, when present as a secondary condition, would be considered a substantial complication or comorbidity—defined as an illness that would increase a length of stay by at least one day for at least 75% of patients.

The MDCs are defined as follows:

1. Diseases and disorders of the nervous system
2. Diseases and disorders of the eye
3. Ear, nose, mouth, throat, and craniofacial diseases and disorders
4. Diseases and disorders of the respiratory system
5. Diseases and disorders of the circulatory system
6. Diseases and disorders of the digestive system
7. Diseases and disorders of the hepatobiliary system and pancreas
8. Diseases and disorders of the musculoskeletal system and connective tissue
9. Diseases and disorders of the skin, subcutaneous tissue, and breast
10. Endocrine, nutritional, and metabolic diseases and disorders
11. Diseases and disorders of the kidney and urinary tract
12. Diseases and disorders of the male reproductive system
13. Diseases and disorders of the female reproductive system
14. Pregnancy, childbirth, and the puerperium
15. Newborns and other neonates with conditions originating in the perinatal period
16. Diseases and disorders of blood, blood forming organs, and immunological disorders
17. Lymphatic, hematopoietic, other malignancies, chemotherapy, and radiotherapy
18. Infectious and parasitic diseases, systemic or unspecified sites
19. Mental diseases and disorders
20. Alcohol/drug use and alcohol/drug induced organic mental disorders
21. Poisonings, toxic effects, other injuries, and other complications of treatment
22. Burns

The evolution of the DRGs and their use as the basic unit of payment in Medicare's hospital reimbursement system represents recognition of the fundamental role of a case mix within a hospital's determination of costs. In the past, hospital characteristics such as teaching status and bed size were used to explain substantial cost differences among hospitals. Such characteristics failed to account adequately for the cost impact of a hospital's case mix. Individual hospitals have often attempted to justify higher cost by contending that they treated a more complex mix of patients. The usual contention was that patients treated by these hospitals were sicker. Although there was a consensus in the hospital industry that a more complex case mix results in higher costs, the concept of case mix complexity had historically lacked a precise definition.

The Concept of Case Mix Complexity

Case mix complexity refers to an interrelated but distinct set of patient attributes, including severity of illness, risk of dying, prognosis, treatment difficulty, need for intervention, and resource intensity. They are defined as follows:

Severity of Illness: Refers to the extent of physiologic decompensation or loss of function in an organ system.

Risk of Mortality: Refers to the likelihood of dying.

Prognosis: Refers to the probable outcome of an illness, including the likelihood of improvement or deterioration in the severity of the illness, recurrence likelihood, and probable life span.

Treatment Difficulty: Refers to the patient management problems which a particular illness presents to the health care provider. Such management problems are associated with illnesses without a clear pattern of symptoms, illnesses requiring sophisticated and technically difficult procedures, and illnesses requiring close monitoring and supervision.

Need for Intervention: Relates to the consequences in terms of severity of illness that lack of immediate or continuing care would produce.

Resource Intensity: Refers to the relative volume and types of diagnostic, therapeutic, and bed services used in the management of a particular illness.

For clinicians, increased case mix complexity refers to greater severity of illness, greater risk of mortality, greater treatment difficulty, poorer prognoses, or a greater need for intervention. Thus, from a clinical perspective, case mix complexity refers to the condition of treated patients and treatment difficulty. Administrators and regulators usually use the concept of case mix complexity to indicate that patients require more resources, resulting in higher costs of care. Thus, from an administrative or regulatory perspective, case mix complexity refers to the resource intensity demands that patients place on an institution. While the two interpretations of case mix complexity are often closely related, they can be very different for certain kinds of patients. For example, while terminal cancer patients are very severely ill and have a high case complexity, they require few hospital resources beyond basic nursing care and are therefore less expensive. No measure of case mix complexity can be equally effective for every aspect.

Patient Classification

Given that the purpose of the DRGs is to relate a hospital's case mix to its resource intensity, it became necessary to develop an operational means of determining patient types and the resources they consumed. While all patients are unique, groups of patients have demographic, diagnostic, and therapeutic attributes in common that determine their level of resource intensity. By developing clinically similar groups of patients with similar resource intensity, patients can be aggregated into meaningful patient groups. Moreover, if these patient groups cover an entire range of patients seen in an inpatient setting, then they would collectively constitute a patient classification scheme that provides a means of establishing and measuring hospital case mix complexity. DRGs were therefore developed as a patient classification scheme consisting of groups of patients who were similar, both clinically, and in terms of their consumption of hospital resources.

Basic Characteristics of the DRG Patient Classification System

Given the limitations of previous patient classification systems and the development of DRGs, it was concluded that in order for the DRG patient classification system to be practical and meaningful, it should have the following characteristics:

- Patient characteristics should be limited to information collected in hospital abstract systems.
- There should be a manageable number of DRGs which encompass all patients seen on an inpatient basis.
- Each DRG should contain patients with a similar pattern of resource intensity.
- Each DRG should contain patients who are similar from a clinical perspective.

Creating DRGs based on information that is collected only in a few settings, or on information that is difficult to collect or measure, would have resulted in a patient classification scheme that could not be applied uniformly across hospitals. This is not to say that information beyond that currently collected might not be useful for defining the DRGs. As additional information becomes routinely available, it must be evaluated to determine if it could result in improvements in the ability to classify patients. Limiting the number of DRGs to manageable numbers ensures that a typical hospital will have enough experience to allow meaningful comparative analysis to be performed. If there were only few patients in each DRG, it would be difficult to detect patterns in case mix complexity and cost performance and to communicate the results to the physician staff. The resource intensity of the patients in each DRG must be similar in order to establish a relationship between the case mix of a hospital and the resources it consumes. When applied properly, the definition of the DRG will not be so specific that every patient is identical, but the level of variation is known and predictable.

Patients in each DRG must be similar from a clinical perspective. In other words, the definition of each DRG must be clinically coherent, requiring patient characteristics to relate to common organ systems or etiologies and that a specific medical specialty should typically provide care to patients. A common organ system or etiology and a common clinical specialty are necessary but not sufficient requirements for a DRG to be clinically coherent. In addition, all available patient characteristics, which medically would be expected to consistently affect resource intensity, should be included in the definition of the DRG. Furthermore, the definition of a DRG should not be based on patient characteristics that medically would not be expected to consistently affect resource intensity.

Major DRG Classifications for Atypical Information

The actual process of forming the DRGs was highly iterative, involving a combination of statistical results from test data with clinical judgment. At any point during the definition of the DRGs, there would often be several patient characteristics which appeared important for understanding the impact on hospital resources.

The selection of the patient characteristics to be used, and the order in which they would be used, was a complex task with many factors examined and weighed simultaneously. The end result of this process was the formation of a comprehensive set of DRGs that described all patients treated in acute care hospitals. There are five DRGs for patients whose medical record abstracts contain clinically atypical or invalid information. They include the following:

- DRG 468 Extensive OR Procedure Unrelated to the Principal Diagnosis
- DRG 476 Prostatic OR Procedure Unrelated to the Principal Diagnosis
- DRG 477 Nonextensive OR Procedure Unrelated to the Principal Diagnosis
- DRG 469 Principal Diagnosis Invalid as Discharge Diagnosis
- DRG 470 Ungroupable

Patients are assigned to DRGs 468, 476, or 477 when all of the operating room (OR) procedures performed are unrelated to the MDCs of the patient's principal diagnosis.

Typically, these are patients admitted for particular diagnoses requiring no surgery, who develop a complication unrelated to the principal diagnosis and who have an OR procedure performed for the complication or for a secondary diagnosis. Unrelated OR procedures have been divided into three groups based on hospital resource use: extensive, prostatic, and nonextensive.

Patients are assigned to DRG 469 when a principal diagnosis is coded which, although it is a valid *ICD-9-CM* code, is not precise enough to allow the patient to be assigned to a clinically coherent DRG. For example, *ICD-9-CM* code 64690 is an unspecified complication of pregnancy with the episode of care unspecified. This diagnosis code does not indicate the type of complication or provide further information about the episode of care. Because DRG definitions assign patients depending on whether the episode of care was antepartum, postpartum, or for delivery, a patient with a principal diagnosis of 64690 will be assigned to DRG 469.

It should be noted that patients with a principal diagnosis not typically considered a reason for hospitalization are not assigned to DRG 469. For example, *ICD-9-CM* code V503, ear piercing, is assigned to DRG 467 and not to DRG 469. Patients are assigned to DRG 470 if certain types of medical record errors are present, which may affect DRG assignment. Patients with an invalid or nonexistent *ICD-9-CM* code as principal diagnosis will be assigned to DRG 470. Patients will also be assigned to DRG 470 if their age, sex, or discharge status is both invalid and necessary for DRG assignment.

Revisions of the DRGs for Medicare

Original DRG definitions were intended to describe each type of patient seen in an acute care hospital. Thus, the DRGs encompassed both the elderly patient population, as well as the newborn, pediatric, and adult populations. With the implementation of the Medicare PPS in 1983, the responsibility for the maintenance and modification of the DRG definitions became the responsibility of the CMS. Since the inception of the Medicare PPS, DRG definitions have been updated annually, although the focus of all modifications has been related to the elderly population.

The health care industry uses DRGs across a wide array of applications: Hospitals have used DRGs for internal management systems, Medicaid programs and Blue Cross plans have used DRGs for payment systems, and state data commissions have used DRGs for statewide comparative reporting systems. Most of these applications have utilized the DRGs across the entire patient population. Thus, the failure of the DRG update process to address problems within non-elderly populations is a serious limitation for most applications.

Major Complications and Comorbidities in AP-DRGs

Some complications and comorbidities (CCs) will have a greater impact on hospital resource use than others. The AP-DRGs designate a subset of the CCs as major CCs. The impact of the presence of major CCs was evaluated for each MDC, and in many cases, their presence had a dominant effect on the resources used by the patient. To avoid significantly increasing the number of DRGs, a single major CC AP-DRG across all surgical patients within an MDC and a single major CC AP-DRG across all medical patients within an MDC were formed for some MDCs.

AP-DRG Hierarchy

The departure in the AP-DRGs from the use of principal diagnosis as the initial variable in DRG assignment made it necessary to form a hierarchy of all exceptions to principal diagnosis based on MDC assignment. For example, based on this hierarchy, if a patient has a tracheostomy and multiple trauma, the patient is assigned to the appropriate tracheostomy AP-DRG.

Pediatric and Other AP-DRG Modifications

The AP-DRGs introduce many other changes to the CMS DRGs. Some of these primarily affect pediatric patients, whereas others affect patients of all ages. The pediatric modifications include some of the recommendations originally developed by the National Association of Children's Hospitals and Related Institutions (NACHRI). In the following areas, either additional AP-DRGs were created or significant modifications were made.

- Pediatric ventricular shunts
- Pediatric cystic fibrosis
- Lead poisoning
- Spinal fusion
- Compulsive nutritional disorders
- Infant aftercare for weight gain
- High-risk obstetric care
- Tertiary aftercare for multiple trauma acute leukemia
- Multiple-channel cochlear implants
- Hemophilia Factor VIII and IX diseases
- Traumatic stupor, coma, concussion, and intracranial injuries
- Bronchopulmonary dysplasia
- Congenital anomalies
- Sickle cell crisis

In addition, AP-DRGs subdivide many of the pediatric groups based on CCs, whereas the CMS DRGs do not. The AP-DRGs also modified many of the basic components of the CMS DRGs. For example, diagnoses were deleted from the CC list, the CC exclusion list was modified, and the surgical hierarchies were modified.

The Development of APR-DRGs: Expanding the Scope of the DRG System

The original objective of the DRGs was to develop a patient classification system that related patient type to resources. The CMS DRGs and AP-DRGs have remained focused on this limited objective, and as a result, there has been increased demand for a patient classification system that can be used for applications beyond resource use, cost, and payment. In particular, a patient classification system is needed for:

- The comparison of hospitals across a wide range of resource and outcome measures. Such comparisons are typically disseminated to the public by state data commissions.
- The evaluation of differences in inpatient mortality rates.
- The implementation and support of critical pathways.
- The identification of continuous quality improvement projects.
- The basis of internal management and planning systems.
- The management of capitated payment arrangements.

APR-DRGs expand the basic DRG structure by adding four subclasses to each DRG, which address patient differences relating to illness severity and mortality risk. Thus, in the APR-DRG system, a patient is assigned three distinct descriptors.

- The base APR-DRG
- The severity of illness subclass
- The risk of mortality subclass

The four severity of illness subclasses and the four risk of mortality subclasses are numbered sequentially from 1 to 4: minor, moderate, major, or extreme severity of illness or risk of mortality. Although categorized numerically, values represent categories and not scores. Thus, it is not meaningful to average the numeric values of illness severity or mortality risk across a group of patients to compute an average severity score. However, the APR-DRG severity and risk of mortality subclasses can be used to compute an expected value for a measure of interest, using statistical techniques such as indirect rate standardization.

The underlying clinical principle of APR-DRGs is that the severity of illness or risk of mortality subclass of a patient is highly dependent on the patient's underlying problem, and that patients with high severity of illness or risk of mortality are usually characterized by multiple serious diseases or illnesses.

The Development Process

The process used in the development of the APR-DRGs involved an iterative process of formulating clinical hypotheses and then testing them against historical data.

Separate clinical models were developed for each of the base APR-DRGs. Once the clinical model for severity of illness and risk of mortality was developed for each base APR-DRG, it was evaluated with historical data in order to review the clinical hypotheses. If there was a discrepancy between clinical expectations and the data results, the clinical content of the *ICD-9-CM* diagnosis and procedure codes was closely examined to determine if ambiguities in the definition or content of the codes could explain the discrepancy. Any discrepancies between clinical expectations and data results were always resolved by using clinical expectations as the basis for the APR-DRGs. Thus, the APR-DRGs are a clinical model that has been extensively tested with historical data. The historical data used in the development of Version 20.0 of the APR-DRGs was a nationwide database of 8.5 million discharges, which included all payer discharges from 1,000 general hospitals from 10 states, and all payer discharges from 47 children's hospitals in the United States.

Development of the Base APR-DRG

The AP-DRGs were initially used as the base DRGs in the formation of the initial APR-DRGs. A series of consolidations, additions, and modifications were then made to these initial APR-DRGs to create the base APR-DRGs. The first step in forming the APR-DRGs was to consolidate all age, CC, and major CC splits. The APR-DRGs also consolidated all splits based on discharge status of death. This was necessary so that death as an outcome variable could be examined across all the APR-DRGs.

In addition to these uniform consolidations, the APR-DRG system introduced an extensive set of consolidations, additions, and refinements to the initial APR-DRG categories. The APR-DRG system has also introduced numerous changes to the definition of MDCs and the pre-MDC hierarchies and categories. Finally, the APR-DRG system has introduced a new kind of logic referred to as *rerouting logic*, which reassigns a patient to a new MDC and APR-DRG in certain circumstances where the principal diagnosis is overly broad or the sequencing of principal and secondary diagnosis is unclear. Altogether, these changes result in a set of base APR-DRGs that are very different from those of other DRG classification systems.

Overview of APR-DRG Subclass Assignment for Secondary Diagnosis

The process of determining the subclasses for an APR-DRG begins by first assigning a severity of illness level and a risk of mortality level to each secondary diagnosis. The term *level* is used when referring to the categorization of a secondary diagnosis. The term *subclass* is used when referring to one of the subdivisions of an APR-DRG. For secondary diagnoses, there are four distinct severity of illness levels and four distinct risk of mortality levels. The four levels are numbered sequentially from 1 to 4 indicating, respectively, minor, moderate, major, or extreme severity of illness or risk of mortality. Each secondary diagnosis is assigned to one of the four severity of illness levels and one of the four risk of mortality levels. The severity of illness level and risk of mortality level associated with a patient's secondary diagnoses is just one factor in the determination of a patient's overall severity of illness subclass and risk of mortality subclass. The assignment of a patient to a severity of illness or risk of mortality subclass takes into consideration not only the level of the secondary diagnoses but also the interaction among secondary diagnoses, age, principal diagnosis, and the presence of certain OR procedures and non-OR procedures.

THE PROCESS OF DETERMINING ILLNESS SEVERITY

There is a three-phase process for determining the severity of illness subclass. There are six steps to Phase I, three steps to Phase II, and nine steps to Phase III for a total of 18 steps.

Phase I—Determine the Severity of Illness Level of Each Secondary Diagnosis

1. Eliminate secondary diagnoses associated with the principal diagnosis. If a secondary diagnosis is closely related to the principal diagnosis and does not add any distinguishing information, the secondary diagnosis is excluded from the determination of the severity of illness subclass.

2. Assign each secondary diagnosis to its standard severity of illness level. Each secondary diagnosis is assigned to one of the four distinct severity of illness levels.

3. Modify the standard severity of illness level of a secondary diagnosis based on age. The age of the patient will modify the standard severity of illness level assignment for some secondary diagnoses.

4. Modify the standard severity of illness level of a secondary diagnosis based on the APR-DRG and principal diagnosis.

5. Modify the standard severity of illness level of a secondary diagnosis based on the APR-DRG. The standard severity of illness level for many secondary diagnoses may be modified depending on the APR-DRG to which the patient is assigned.

6. Modify the standard severity of illness level of a secondary diagnosis based on non-OR procedures.

Phase II—Determine the Base Severity of Illness Subclass for the Patient

Once each secondary diagnosis has been assigned its standard severity of illness level and the standard severity of illness level of each secondary diagnosis has been modified based on age, APR-DRG and principal diagnosis, APR-DRG, and presence of certain non-OR procedures, the Phase II base severity of illness subclass for the patient can be determined. The process of determining the base patient severity of illness subclass of the patient begins with the elimination of certain secondary diagnoses that are closely related to other secondary diagnoses. The elimination of these diagnoses prevents the double counting of clinically similar diagnoses in the determination of the severity of illness subclass of the patient. Once redundant diagnoses have been eliminated, the base severity of illness subclass is determined based on all of the remaining secondary diagnoses. There are three steps to Phase II.

1. Eliminate certain secondary diagnoses from the determination of the severity of illness subclass of the patient. Closely related secondary diagnoses are grouped together with clinically similar diagnoses. If more than one secondary diagnosis from the same secondary diagnosis group is present, then only the secondary diagnosis with the highest severity of illness level is preserved. All other secondary diagnoses in the group have their severity

level reduced to minor, virtually eliminating them from contributing to the patient's base subclass determination.

2. Combine all secondary diagnoses to determine the base severity of illness subclass of the patient. Once secondary diagnoses that are related to other secondary diagnoses have had their severity levels reduced to minor, the base patient severity of illness subclass is set equal to the maximum severity of illness level across all of the remaining secondary diagnoses.

3. Reduce the base severity of the patient illness subclass with a major or extreme subclass unless the patient has multiple secondary diagnoses at a high severity level. In order to be assigned to the major or extreme severity of illness subclass, a patient must have multiple secondary diagnoses at a high severity of illness level.

Phase III—Determine the Final Severity of Illness Subclass of the Patient

Once the base patient severity of illness subclass is computed, the patient severity of illness subclass may be increased or decreased based on specific values of the following patient attributes:

- Combinations of APR-DRG and principal diagnosis
- Combinations of APR-DRG and age, or APR-DRG and principal diagnosis and age
- Combinations of APR-DRG and non-OR procedures
- Combinations of APR-DRG and OR procedures
- Combinations of APR-DRG and pairs of OR procedures
- Combination of APR-DRG for extracorporeal membrane oxygenation (ECMO) and presence/absence of certain OR procedures
- Combinations of APR-DRG and principal diagnoses and non-OR procedures
- Combinations of categories of secondary diagnoses

Phase III examines these eight patient attributes, seven of which are APR-DRG specific, and then as its ninth step, computes the patient's final severity of illness subclass assignment. Then, complete the following steps:

1. Modify severity of illness subclass for the patient based on combinations of APR-DRG and principal diagnosis. This step is used extensively in Phase III to modify a patient's severity of illness subclass. The *ICD-9-CM* coding system will sometimes include in a single diagnosis code both the underlying disease and an associated manifestation of the disease.

2. Modify severity of illness subclass for the patient based combinations of APR-DRG and age or APR-DRG, principal diagnosis, and age. For some principal diagnoses in specific APR-DRGs, the patient's age essentially represents a complicating factor. For specific principal diagnoses and age combinations in certain APR-DRGs, the severity of illness subclass of the patient is increased by a specified increment up to a specified maximum subclass.

3. Modify the severity of illness subclass for the patient based on combinations of APR-DRG and non-OR procedures. For some APR-DRGs, the presence of certain non-OR procedures represents a complicating factor.

4. Modify the severity of illness subclass for the patient based on combinations of APR-DRG and OR procedure.

5. Modify the severity of illness subclass for the patient based on combinations of APR-DRG and pairs of OR procedures.

6. Modify the severity of illness subclass for the patient based on combination of APR-DRG for ECMO and presence/absence of certain OR procedures.

7. Modify the severity of illness subclass for the patient based on combinations of APR-DRG, principal diagnosis, and non-OR procedure.

8. Establish a minimum severity of illness subclass for the patient based on the presence of specific combinations of categories of secondary diagnoses.

9. Compute the final patient severity of illness subclass (Averill et al., 2003, pp. 1–62).

To be fully reimbursed for hospital care provided, it is essential to understand the difference between Medicare and Medicaid and their characteristics. Discharge data sets for your hospital must be uniform to avoid possible complications. Understanding of the DRGs, from its history to the concept of case mix complexity will help you classify patients correctly. Ideally, reimbursement for patient services should be clear and efficient. By avoiding mistakes and assigning proper DRGs, your department will be appropriately reimbursed for the level of care provided.

MANAGED CARE CONTRACTS

A great deal of attention is focused on reimbursement for patient stays, which relates to government reimbursement by way of DRGs and the ongoing attention of health care reform and reductions in reimbursements from the CMS. It is important to also understand how managed care contracts through commercial payers affect patient care. These locally negotiated contracts for patient payments impact budgets, the patient length of stay, and resource consumption.

Managed Care 101

Managed care is an evolving nomenclature that continues to transform into various hybrids. However, the foundation remains the same, it is a system designed to control medical costs by allowing only medically necessary health care services to be provided to a patient in the most cost-effective setting.

Over the years, managed care has mutated from small and narrow health maintenance organization (HMO) networks to large and expanded preferred provider organization (PPO) networks as consumers demanded choice and open access. The open access or PPO networks were created out of consumer demand for choice.

Recent arrangements, such as health savings accounts, are designed to involve consumers in their health care decision-making process by enticing them to choose the most cost effective, highest quality physician and hospital to provide the services. Still, health care is one of the only commodities purchased by consumers where the cost is unknown until after the fact.

Managed Care Contracting 101

The scope of contract review should be rigorous and detailed to evaluate the overall cost benefit of the relationship. The goal is to create a working document that both parties can abide by for the duration of the contract period. The contract is much more than reimbursement; it is a living, breathing document. Adding language that protects the organization from risk is a serious responsibility and one that should not be taken lightly.

The managed care or legal department can negotiate language modifications in an effort to create a mutually beneficial contract. The more leverage a provider has in a market helps, although smaller operations can succeed in obtaining a reciprocal contract that will help protect assets.

The execution of the contract is only the beginning; the operational aspects of the relationship are crucial in making certain the parties are meeting their contractual obligations. Establishing a Joint Operations Committee (JOC) meeting monthly or quarterly is extremely beneficial to keep the parties on track and focused. The meetings address any accounts receivable issues such as slow pay, short pays, or other claim trends. Additionally, the meetings address any case management or denial issues. Generally speaking, matters can be resolved amicably and within a reasonable amount of time. The JOCs are most successful when executive-level leadership involvement on both sides are involved.

Creating a report including various statistics regarding the payer's performance such as timely payment, grievances and appeals, denials that are overturned in the providers favor, and so forth is a tool that can be used and reviewed for contract evaluation purposes. The goal is to capture trends to determine the "red tape" analysis with the relationship.

Reimbursement 101

The reimbursement structure for a hospital is dependent on business strategy and high-volume service lines. Reimbursement methodologies come in many different shapes and sizes from per diems (a set per day amount paid for each day a patient is in the hospital) to a DRG. Case rate carve outs that are similar to DRG payments, however, can also have a length of stay limit for which a hospital would get an additional payment or per diem for every day the patient is in house beyond the threshold set for the length of stay.

A good gauge of how an organization would perform under any methodology is to test the population against varying rate structures. Another basic test to evaluate the hospital's length of stay is to compare it to the Medicare's geometric mean length of stay (an allotted time calculated for a typical patient stay in the hospital). Other examples of key measures are to determine if the net revenue is per discharge and per day by DRG and service lines.

One of the keys to successful negotiation is to know what the long-term business line strategy is of a hospital.

Contract Language Review 101

Policies and Procedures

A payer's base agreement is typically structured to benefit the payer and not the provider. In general, the contract will contain language that requires the provider to abide by and be bound to all of the payer guidelines, metrics, and administrative policies and procedures. The contracts usually have a provision stating that the payer can change his or her policies at any time without prior approval by the provider.

There is contractual language that allows a hospital to terminate a contract as well. This language refers to when a material change occurs to their policies that negatively impacts a hospital financially or operationally. Given such a situation, at minimum, a hospital should have an opportunity to reevaluate the financial terms of an agreement. To be clear, however, ensure that policies "attached hereto and incorporated herein" are thoroughly reviewed by leaders in the various segments of a hospital.

Note as well that these sections in the contract are often greater in scope than one would think. For example, there are requirements for the provider to submit copies of entire medical records, which is extremely costly and laborious. A remedy exists, however, at least in blunting the impact of the volume and costs of such requests by charging the payer a per page amount for copies.

In addition, make certain that the provider has adequate appeal rights for denials or payment reductions caused by lack of preauthorization, level of care, length of stay, and/or medical necessity, which are the most common reasons why a provider is at risk for a payer recouping funds.

Utilization Review/Case Management

In light of recent focus on one-day stays and levels of care, a provider should be resolute in adding contract language that mitigates his or her risk for nonpayment or short payment. Any disagreement between the payer and provider, as it relates to level of care or length of stay, should be addressed and resolved while the patient is in the hospital. A swift resolution will alleviate the backlog of denials and appeals. It will provide both parties the opportunity to discuss the details of the case and then make a determination real time, rather than waiting until after the patient has been discharged. This typically is done via the concurrent review process that can be performed either on site or by telephone, depending on patient volumes. To avoid a backlog of disputes, a provider can negotiate language that requires the payer to notify the provider prior to recouping funds, short paying a stay, or denying it in its entirety. The key here is to prevent the payer from having the right to short pay or deny the entire stay as he or she wishes.

It is typical for the commercial sector to follow the footsteps of CMS. They will begin to use any guidelines they can to deny the stay or conduct audits and recoup payments made for 1-day stays. The case management department, in conjunction with physician and administrative leadership teams, must be on the same page with criteria used to measure the appropriateness of the stay.

Member and Provider

Language pertaining to membership is also important. The provider should have 24-hour availability to the payer in order to verify patient's eligibility, benefits, and to obtain prior authorizations or to notify the plan of services rendered. Be aware of the retroactive eligibility shortfall. Typically, the contract will allow the payer to go back as far as he or she needs to when recouping dollars for services rendered to a member who was ineligible at the time of service. The time frame for retroactive eligibility refunds should be reasonably limited to 6 months, for example.

As it relates to members, the provider should always insist on a provision in the contract that allows him or her to collect co-pays, coinsurance, and deductibles *at the time of service*. The likelihood of collecting the full amount for high-dollar cases from a patient afterward is dramatically reduced.

A common term is *bad debt*, which refers to an amount owed that is written off because the debt is unable to be collected, and all reasonable efforts to collect the debt have been exhausted. As more benefit plans require a greater out-of-pocket expense from members, providers experience a greater impact of bad debt, meaning that the price negotiated for the service is not being paid in full. To avoid the downward spiral of these incidents, a provider can work with the payer to negotiate a threshold of reasonable bad debt for the provider. Negotiating increased rates is one method of offsetting bad debt.

Claims Processing, Timely Filing, and Refunds

The agreement should clearly specify the time when the plan is allotted to approve or deny claims and make payment. This is recommended even if state law addresses the issue because some state statutes allow the parties to contract for a different time. Additionally, some states do not define a "clean claim," allowing the plan to avoid the provision for prompt payment.

The issue of timely payment—a steady stream of cash—is vital to a business' success. Therefore, the provider should insist that a payer reimburse the provider for services within 30 days of the provider's submission of a "clean claim," which can loosely be defined as a claim that does not require additional information, void of coding, or billing errors.

There should be protection for the provider if the payer fails to abide by timely payment. Many states already require that interest be applied to the claim if payment is not timely received. If one's state does not have prompt payment protection, other tactics may include reverting to 100% of billed charges if the claim is not paid within the specified time frame, or some sort of an interest or cash payment penalty for repeated incidents for late or partial payments.

If the payer requires additional information for a claim submitted, the payer should provide written notice to the provider of any alleged deficiencies in any submitted claim within a reasonable amount of time, such as 10 days after receipt of such claim.

In terms of timely billing for the provider, the preferred standard should be any state or federal requirements. In lieu of established guidelines, a longer time to submit claims from provider to payer is best. Payers should not be given carte blanche— the right to recoup or offset payments to the provider without written notice to the provider—as well as giving the provider adequate time to review the request to determine if he or she agrees with the refund request. It is up to an organization's policies to clarify issues related to erroneous amounts paid. This is especially true in terms of an offset of future claims for unrelated cases or the distribution of cash for erroneous amounts paid. Be certain to limit the time for such recoveries to 1 year; otherwise, a hospital could be asked to refund dollars for a case that is several years old. In addition, this provision should be reciprocal.

Legal Provisions

Every payer requires general and professional liability insurance, and rightly so. Verify that each party is responsible for its own costs and that the organization meets the standards contractually required, particularly if an organization is self-insured.

The assignment clause is something that is often overlooked. This section is typically one sided, allowing only the payer to assign or delegate duties. This section should be reciprocal, so that neither party can assign duties without consent of the other party.

The ability to market and promote the provider is essential when working with any payer. Most agreements include a provision that allows the payer to publish information about the provider to the public. This is great for business development and exposure; however, make sure that any direct advertising piece, including information other than generic location and contact information, is reviewed prior to publication for accuracy. Also, the agreement should not require the provider to participate in all products offered or administered by the payer as a condition of participating in any individual plan or plans. This should be mutually negotiated between the parties.

Most organizations have attorneys review the entire contract. Have legal counsel lend their expertise to provisions such as arbitration, indemnification, grievance, appeals, and coordination of benefits. The key to these sections involves ensuring that each party is financially responsible for their own acts and omissions. Parties should have the opportunity to resolve issues via an appeals and grievance process prior to arbitration, mediation, or court proceeding.

It is perfectly acceptable and practical to enter into multiple-year payer contracts. Not only because it takes several months to determine the legal and financial terms of an agreement, but also payers require network stability for their sales efforts.

The reality is that entering into a payer contract is the same as entering into any business relationship. There must be transparency and mutual benefits. If these basic fundamental components are not established from the beginning then both parties are looking at a long and potentially rocky relationship.

SUMMARY

Managed care contracts impact budget, length of stay, and resource consumption. By allowing only the necessary procedures to be performed, they reduce costs and ensure patient quality of care. The transformation of HMOs to PPOs provides a working document that not only reimburses the hospital but also protects your department from unnecessary risk. By being familiar with reimbursement methods and basic contract terminology you will be able to create managed care contracts that increase department efficiency and reduce possible complications.

NOTE

1. Used with permission from 3M, the discussion provided on pages 105–115 on the patient classification scheme, drug-related diagnosis, is derived from a pdf titled, All-Patient Refined Diagnosis Related Groups (APR-DRGs), Version 20.0, Methodology Overview, written by Richard F. Averill, Norbet Goldfield, MD, Jack S. Hughes, MD, Janice Bonazelli, Elizabeth C. McCullough, Barbara A. Steinbeck, Robert Mullin, MD, and Ana M. Tang of 3M; John Muldoon and Lisa Turner of the National Association of Children's Hospitals and Related Institutions, Inc.; and James Gay, MD, of the Medical Advisory Committee for NACHRI APR-DRG Research Project, Copyright © 2003, 3M. All rights reserved.

Conclusion

Nancy Bateman and Jacklyn Mead

The finance section was designed to provide an overview of financial reporting, finance functions, managing a budget, and defending it when necessary. The section also reviewed how health care is paid for based on provided services. In summary, it is important for one to reach out to one's finance department and care management staff—appreciate the complex world of coding and ask for assistance from the health information management department when questions arise or changes are requested. The basic accounting concepts reviewed in this section provide a good foundation for working within a financially sound department. Using common financial statements and terms provide the cornerstone of budget creation, which results in an accountable, sound outlook on future expenses. Understanding the finance department's role in purchasing allows Nurse Managers to further assure spending compliance and maximum reimbursements. Knowing the difference between governmental and commercial insurance will also ensure that coding adheres to the diagnosis-related group (DRG) payment system structure when reporting elements that concern diagnosis and procedures. Finally, with an overview of the commercial side of reimbursement through managed care contracts your understanding of how to run a department from the business side of nursing will support a fiscally well-run department.

Resource Management

Nancy Bateman

Resource management combines labor and nonlabor resources, applying both components to each encounter during a patient's stay. Referred to as *episodes of care* (EOC), a patient's care is mapped from admission through discharge, with the flow of care broken down into segments. Although labor and nonlabor are analyzed separately, they have a profound influence on one another, focusing attention on the providers of care as well as the supplies and services used. As a manager, it is important to look at each EOC to determine whether the right skill sets and supplies/interventions are available for care. Part IV provides you with the information and the processes you need to deliver the highest quality of care at the lowest cost. It will help you identify any inconsistencies between patient needs and services provided. Throughput, although a difficult process, is essential with the increasing levels of uninsured patients. The three areas to examine when considering throughput are described clearly to allow ease of resource management. Six Sigma, a way to track ongoing compliance, is reviewed in Chapter 9. Do note that tracking is essential for improving performance and maintaining sustainability. Case studies are provided to demonstrate real-life situations where your knowledge will be indispensible.

8

Care Delivery Techniques for High Quality With Low Costs

Nancy Bateman

Throughput and patient flow are often referred to as resource management. The Institute for Healthcare Improvement (http://www.ihi.org) defines *throughput* as the number of health care admissions, including observations, per week. What used to be capacity or medical management has broadened to include effective use of staff, supplies, and services for each episode of patient care. The key to successful improvements in this area is to staff based on demand, monitoring patient demand on a daily basis. In order to sustain these processes, significant improvements are required in labor levels, skill mix alignment with tasks, appropriate use of supplies and services, and care management from patient contact through discharge. This chapter examines the three areas of throughput as well as the various subgroups and parameters for case management.

LEARNING OBJECTIVES

1. Define what resource management is and how it provides a comprehensive view of labor, skills, and supplies.
2. List the subcommittees involved in resource management and their roles in the process.
3. Articulate the importance of process mapping patient encounters.

RESOURCE MANAGEMENT

Resource management in selected services (such as cardiology, cancer, and critical care) provides a competitive advantage as hospital customers, physicians, patients, and staff will be inclined to leave institutions without adequate staffing. Staying within budget and providing the best outcomes possible for patients requires a complete view of their care. Capacity optimization—a metric by which staff levels are matched to patient demand—improves gross sales as other initiatives seek to reduce costs. On average, 35% or more of every additional revenue dollar produced by way of maximizing existing capacity can directly affect hospital profits.

The Elements of Resource Management

Using existing staff efficiently, with less variation of practice and smoother transitions between providers, produces fewer errors and increases patient care. Improved throughput—patient movement in a hospital—can also improve efficiency while reducing costs. Capacity and growth management offer opportunities to improve operating margins: for a typical $1 billion organization, benefits can range from $11.5 to $22 million in capacity, efficiency, and growth-related opportunities. The breakdown of these benefits is length of stay (LOS) reduction resulting in savings of $4.5 to $9 million, improved patient processes for savings of $1 to $2 million, and better management of staff requirements (reduced overtime and agency staff) for another $1 to $2 million in savings.

Resource management uses several elements to achieve this efficiency. First, it builds on the staffing models introduced earlier in this book, assessing needed skills for specific patient needs and tasks. Matching clinical staff resources to demand, although difficult during staffing shortages, is critical to managing costs and staff satisfaction. One of the main reasons for using agency, traveler, and temporary employees is the perception that additional staff is needed, when in fact the full amount of needed staff may already be available if tasks are delegated properly. The need to establish segment-based skill levels is critical in adjusting delegation of duties with current staff.

Second, resource management reviews the pattern in which patients move through departments during their hospital stays. Measured by LOS, each type of patient condition comes with an expected number of hospitalization days. In conjunction with LOS data, throughput assesses the methods by which a patient enters a hospital for care; patients entering a hospital based on physician referral or emergency departments (EDs), for example, receive different orders for care. When these elements are taken into consideration, hospitals can better manage the processes by which they admit and track patients. If patients remain hospitalized for longer than expected, throughput assessment can help diagnose these issues and prevent them from decreasing the institution's profit margin.

A third element in resource management is medical management. Evidence-based medicine (EBM) allows tests and medication orders to be based on proven clinical outcomes. EBM applies the best and most up-to-date information to support medical decision making, assessing the risks and rewards of treatment. Patient care costs can rise considerably if excessive testing or treatments are ordered and do not support improved outcomes.

Finally, the accurate use of patient supplies can reduce costs in nonlabor expenses and help the financial state of a hospital. Both vendor and supply variation reduction can improve quality and outcomes of patient care delivery.

Case Example: Patient Process Flow Mapping

The accurate use of supplies and services promotes consistency of care, improved outcomes, and reduced costs. Process mapping can provide a glimpse into required services and supplies used by an individual patient. Figure 8.1 provides an example process flow for a patient undergoing an elective procedure. (Note: This example is based on a British hospital's work and may therefore reference differing procedural steps to those used within a hospital in the United States.)

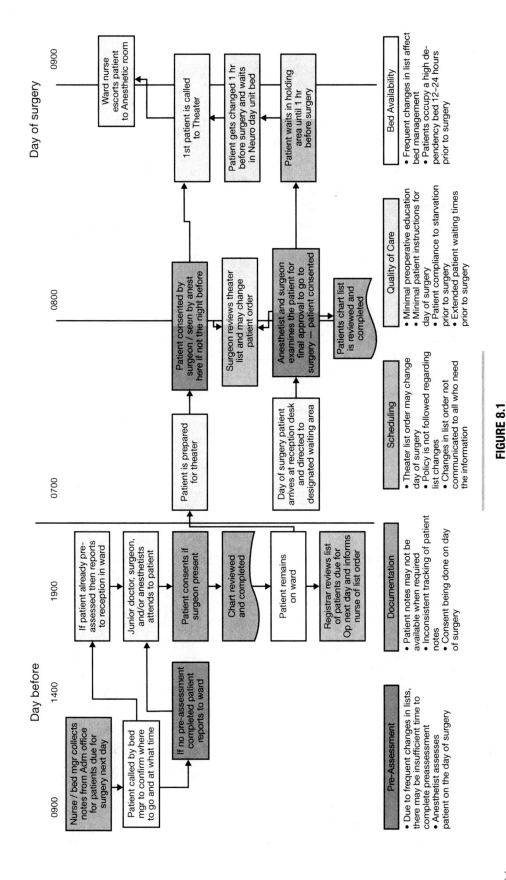

FIGURE 8.1
Day of Surgery Admission Process Map
Current State

127

Once the process map is re-created with the future state flows, it is then expanded to showcase the new patient flow. A future state "Day of Surgery" flow is shown in Figures 8.2 and 8.3.

In addition to a process map, it is useful to create a spreadsheet accounting for medical supplies, organized by their appropriate segment of care. In an EBM approach, assigning supplies can help determine the best use of resources for quality outcomes. Policies and orders may indicate that specific items should be used. Once the parameters of a product are determined, it is then up to materials management to contract for the best price and most comprehensive coverage.

Such a linear approach to delivering care can be separated by episode of care that allows patient care providers to assign skills, services, and supplies to each episode. *The right skill at the right time, with the right supplies and coordination, equals consistent, high-quality care at lower costs.*

Care Pathways and Care Roadmaps

The linear approach is best used with existing care pathways or care roadmaps because they predefine expected LOS and costs of care. Following patient diagnoses as defined in major diagnostic categories (MDCs) and diagnosis-related groups (DRGs) allow patients to receive uniform care and allow hospitals to maximize their insurance reimbursement.

Building extended care pathways with a combination of nonlabor cost management and labor alignment creates high-quality outcomes with reduced variation in treatment. When care pathways are created, LOSs are reduced because staff members understand their roles, work tasks, and expected time lines. Care pathways first gained popularity in the 1970s but waned in use until the health care community became interested in Six Sigma principles to track progress and compliance. Most hospitals now employ at least one black belt, Six Sigma–trained, full-time employee.

Care pathways are designed by a multidisciplinary team of physicians, nurses, social workers, and ancillary support staff using EBM practices. When these pathways are used, assigned tasks are structured to provide clinical appropriateness, clinical effectiveness, and operational effectiveness. Staff satisfaction increases because of confidence in patient care delivery, patient satisfaction increases because of shorter delays and operational competency, families are able to ask more questions to more caregivers about their loved ones' treatment, and physicians appreciate improvements in the structure and improved patient flow. An added value to this approach is the incorporation of wellness efforts, promoting health and optimal patient outcomes as an integral component of the care pathway.

DETERMINING EFFECTIVE PATIENT THROUGHPUT USING PROCESS MAPS

The throughput process can be difficult to manage because of the growing ranks of uninsured patients within the United States receiving primary care in overtaxed EDs. There is a growing mismatch between patient needs and the services available at facilities. As a result of excess capacity, policies and procedures regarding appropriate and efficient deployment of resources have slipped, and technology aimed at managing patient overages has been inconsistently deployed, often resulting in

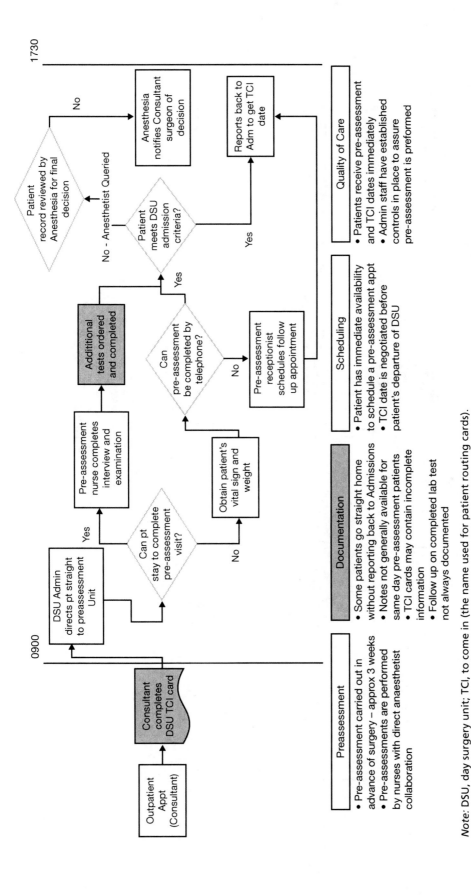

FIGURE 8.2

Day of Surgery Unit Preassessment Unit Process Map Future State

Note: DSU, day surgery unit; TCI, to come in (the name used for patient routing cards).

129

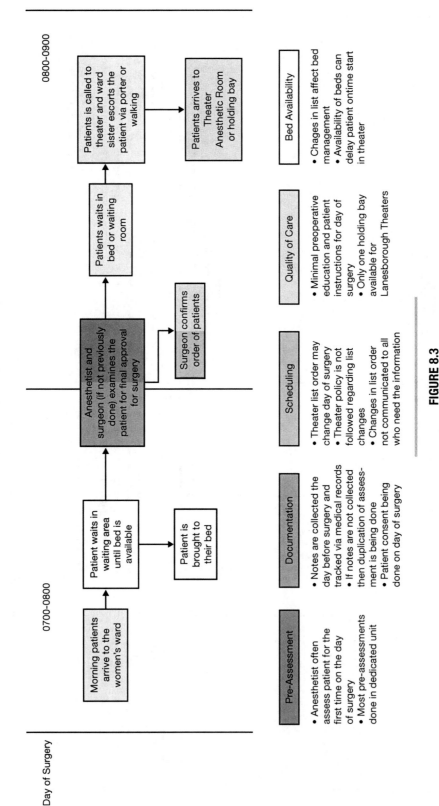

FIGURE 8.3
Day of Surgery Admission Process Map

cumbersome and inefficient systems. Despite the advent of electronic medical records, the interface systems between admissions, patient care, materials management, and specialty departments often lack the ability to share information in real-time basis. Another roadblock impacting throughput is inadequate community health system support, including subacute, long-term care and social services.

Determining if an organization has effective patient throughput requires DRG-based analysis of average LOS and cost. This analysis is commonly tracked by the finance department and begins with performance benchmarking against peer facilities. Common comparatives used include bed size, case mix index, academic versus community hospital designation, as well as other factors that provide a sufficient number of peer facilities. When peer performances are reviewed against your current performance target, improvement goals of LOS and costs can be developed. The next steps are to create work plans to reach targets and meet effective patient throughput using MDCs as your guides. Figure 8.4 exemplifies an analysis of LOS per MDC.

In Figure 8.4 the facility has an opportunity to reduce their LOS across several diagnostic categories. To do so, hospital administrators should compare the costs of care by MDC. The same databases can align this information as shown in Figure 8.5.

Following the two points of reference within Figures 8.4 and 8.5, it is then necessary to prioritize which categories are addressed first. In this scenario, the LOS and costs per case can be brought together, determining that the first three opportunities for DRG savings are related to medical pneumonia (respiratory MDC), cardiac services (circulatory MDC), and total joints (musculoskeletal MDC). This decision can be made partly due to the availability of solid literature and practice patterns aimed

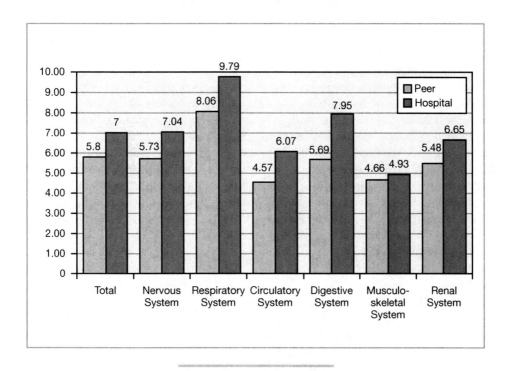

FIGURE 8.4
Sample Length of Stay by MDC

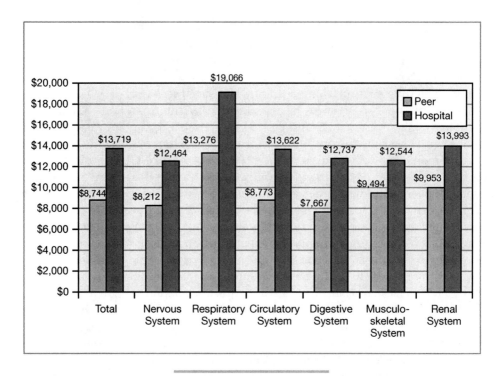

FIGURE 8.5
Sample Cost per Case by MDC

at standardizing order sets within these areas. Another advantage comes in the form of cooperation from various physician groups, including cardiologists, cardiovascular surgeons, orthopedic surgeons, and referring physicians. Once these specialties participated in the process, subsequent DRGs could make use of the same or similar physician groups, allowing for faster and easier outcomes. Once the selected DRGs are identified, complete a process map for DRGs by following selected patients from participating physicians. Process maps define how patient flow is working, comparing current processes to ideal movement. Once the ideal process map is developed, assign staff with the right skills, services, and supplies to each episode of care to complete the process. The latter portion of this chapter revisits this process, including Six Sigma principles in order to track compliance and initiate corrective actions when necessary.

Approach and Methodology

Developing and implementing resource management begins with the assembly of a team of multidisciplinary caregivers that includes all aspects of treatment and services. This is a large group and should be divided by tasks according to the DRG. Team members incorporated into various subgroups include case managers, social workers, bed management staff, selected physicians, surgical services and ED nurses, registration and scheduling staff, finance staff, information technology staff, and representation from the ancillary departments of laboratory, radiology, pharmacy, housekeeping, and therapies. The overall group is large, but there are members such

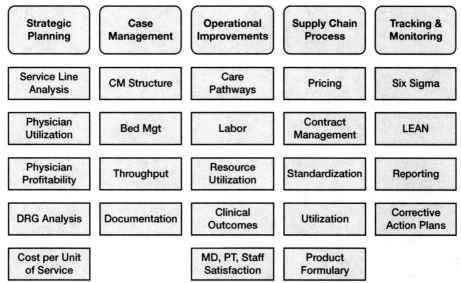

Strategic Planning	Case Management	Operational Improvements	Supply Chain Process	Tracking & Monitoring
Service Line Analysis	CM Structure	Care Pathways	Pricing	Six Sigma
Physician Utilization	Bed Mgt	Labor	Contract Management	LEAN
Physician Profitability	Throughput	Resource Utilization	Standardization	Reporting
DRG Analysis	Documentation	Clinical Outcomes	Utilization	Corrective Action Plans
Cost per Unit of Service		MD, PT, Staff Satisfaction	Product Formulary	

Note: DRG, diagnosis-related group; CM, case management; MD, medical doctor; PT, patient.

FIGURE 8.6
Strategic Planning Subgroup

as nurses and case managers who will be core members, and should participate in the entire process, whereas other members of subgroups attend when their sections are under review or approval for next steps are required.

Whereas each DRG has an assembled team to map future state process flows, care pathways, order sets, and alignment of labor and nonlabor, the oversight team is also segmented into subgroups. Each subgroup meets biweekly, spending their non-meeting weeks advancing the throughput process. The subgroups and their respective responsibilities for outcomes are shown in Figure 8.6.

Strategic Planning Subgroup
Based on the subgroups shown earlier, the strategic planning subgroup is responsible for assisting with service line analysis and physician profitability. Membership in this subgroup is mostly from finance and should include a representative from administration, preferably a CFO or COO. This subgroup can assess and identify high-cost, extended LOS DRGs and perform physician profitability. As the multidisciplinary team meets (representatives from each of the subgroups), the strategic planning subgroup supports the process by reevaluating and performing analysis of the recommended changes to ensure the other team's work is progressing to an improved financial outcome.

Case Management Subgroup
The case management subgroup is responsible for assessing throughput, improving bed management, educating health care providers on appropriate DRG documentation, and garnering correct reimbursements. Combined with their traditional roles, the case management subgroup evaluates current functions as they implement new

models. Revising their services to support the new process care pathways will be a vital part of the sustained success of the models as they are the link between services and patient care needs. A successful care management program reduces variation in practice and reduces days of care for selected medical conditions.

The goal of an effective case management program is to ensure that care is coordinated and seamless while reducing costs through efficient use of resources. Case managers are the facilitators of care. Medical necessity on admission is reviewed by the case manager, and the appropriate documentation to support the level of care is the responsibility of the case manager regardless of the entry point or payer. All too often, case managers review only Medicare patients—and although these cases are important to review, a case manager should also be aware of the different managed-care contracts in use and the specific requirements of each.

The case management model should be unit based or disease based. Case management resources should be provided 7 days a week for all admitted and observation patients. The focus of the model is on interdisciplinary collaboration, ensuring appropriate transitions between all levels of care and includes key linkages to payers and hospitals. A successful operating model improves processes and communication between payers, physicians, and nurses regarding concurrent review and discharge planning. An important component to the model and one which should be enhanced through the resource management process is consistent, timely, and appropriate physician support, as well as timely resolutions to clinical care coordination issues between nursing and physicians.

The Five Performance Parameters of Case Management
Case management includes five performance parameters or areas of focus: quality of care, clinical appropriateness, clinical effectiveness, and patient and family satisfaction. If a facility's model has not progressed from the role of utilization management and there is no representation across all areas, the facility needs to establish a robust program before a full resource management process can be started. The key players in a case management program are program managers, case managers, social workers, physician advisors (PAs), and case management assistants. The program should be operational 7 days a week, with on-site staffing requirements matching periods of high-patient volume. Case managers may be on call for weekend access only as required and staffed appropriately for Monday morning reviews of patients admitted over weekends. All patients should have some form of chart review within 48 hours of admission.

Program Managers
The program manager is responsible for implementing a case management program consistent with an organization's vision and goals. Program managers work collaboratively with PAs and key physicians to ensure attainment of program goals and objectives, creating, implementing, and reviewing program policies and procedures. Whereas the case management assistant will measure and monitor key performance indicators (KPIs), the program manager communicates results to physicians and other leaders and uses results to continuously improve the program. The program manager oversees selection, supervision, and performance appraisal of all clinical care coordination staff, developing and implementing initial and ongoing training and education, and representing the department at meetings with other entities.

Case Managers

The case manager provides coordination of care for patients across the continuum. The current model, unlike older utilization review responsibilities, calls for an integrated role including care coordination, utilization management, and discharge planning. Case managers should have a case load of approximately 1:25 to 30 patients. An important part of the case management process is coordinated handoffs for efficient and effective patient care. A case manager screens all admissions for clinical appropriateness while monitoring resource utilization and performing patient stay reviews.

Case manager qualifications call for candidates to be registered nurses, with more than two years experience in clinical, utilization management, discharge planning, home health care, or ambulatory services. The position demands excellent interpersonal communication and negotiation skill because a case manager liaises with physicians, outside services, and nursing care departments. In a unit-based model, candidates should also possess competence in the appropriate area of work. The position requires strong organizational and time management skills with an ability to work independently.

Social Workers

Social workers compliment the model's different needs by providing psychosocial intervention, crisis intervention, and the mobilization of community resources, with typical case loads of 1:40 to 60 patients. The role supports patients throughout multiple levels of care while helping to obtain access to appropriate resources, ensuring patients are ready for discharge. Social workers may be called on to initiate referrals to protective services in cases of suspected abuse or neglect and may serve as consultants in guardianship, power of attorney, adoption, health care surrogate, and advance directive issues. Qualifications for the social worker require a master's degree in social work (MSW), with referenced clinical competence in the assigned area.

Physician Advisor

The PA provides case management departments with case expertise, staff support, and liaison functions within an organization. The physician (or physicians) occupying this role will review selected cases for the appropriateness of admission, level of care criteria, continuing stay evaluation, and denied cases. PAs act as a resource for medical necessity secondary reviews and observation status discussions. In addition, the PA will facilitate communication and problem resolution with attending physicians.

PA qualifications call for state-licensed medical doctors with staff privileges in an acute in-patient facility; a working knowledge of regulatory, payer, and utilization management issues; and a commitment to the organization's vision, goals, and objectives for care management. It is highly beneficial if the PA has recognition by his or her peers as an outstanding clinician and a proven capability to communicate with physician colleagues. The PA must also demonstrate consistent objectivity, flexibility, and tact in dealing with potentially sensitive staff issues, practice patterns, and clinical resource utilization. Additional education and experience in the areas of case management, utilization management, and quality improvement is a great addition to the position.

Case Manager Assistant

The final position is the case manager assistant, which provides support for case managers within the system by communicating with payers on simple cases; assists with denial management; arranges simple, nonacute, postdischarge services; and performs administrative and secretarial duties.

Physician Component

The physician component to throughput improvements depends on their behaviors and practice patterns because this impacts the ability to move patients in an efficient and cost-effective manner. Delayed throughput is often caused by lack of knowledge or access to admission criteria for specific inpatient units, resulting in inappropriate placement or failure to place patients in an appropriate level of care. Patients cannot be discharged in a timely manner if discharge orders are not written or if physicians are not responsive after receiving test results. These issues can be addressed by medical directors and hospitalist programs facilitating compliance with admission and discharge criteria while providing oversight. During implementation of the revised care pathways, educational programs on evidence-based admission and discharge criteria should be incorporated into the process. A communication model for physicians is vital for successful implementation.

Bed Placement

A part of throughput is bed placement; plans should be created with a clinical approach, tracking where beds are and how they will be allocated. Map out each department using the average daily census, historical trending, and current physician mix to estimate future needs as units may need to shift their allocation of beds. Before the end of the project, a clinical resource management program should be created to continue work across the next level of DRGs in the prioritized list. For this reason, the case management program will be an extended and highly visible subset of the new program.

Tracking and Monitoring

Within the overall project, the tracking and monitoring subgroup is responsible for monitoring outcomes and initiative corrective action plans when compliance or variations outside approved levels occur. A case manager is an extended team member, contributing his or her to help develop tools and establish variance levels. Case managers are also in an ideal position to monitor concurrent reviews of patient charts and should review ongoing physician documentation to educate and remind physicians of proper documentation for treatment plans because they affect reimbursement and patient care. It is important not only for physicians to document their test result reviews and alterations to treatment plans, but to also add documentation as necessary. Coders in medical records cannot adjust DRG levels without proper physician notation, making this element of care essential for billing and efficiency purposes.

Most hospitals have tackled throughput at one time or another and the issue poses a continuing struggle even when programs are already in place. There are three areas to examine regarding throughput. Figure 8.7 demonstrates typical questions as they arise within the stages of patient throughput.

The case management team, working in collaboration with nurses, physicians, and administrators, should attempt to answer the questions earlier, reviewing data needed to assess each aspect of throughput. Once the current state is effectively assessed, a corrective work plan can be developed.

Access	Throughput	Disposition
• Are there issues with bed management/assignment, e.g. saturation, unavailability?	• Can orders be initiated immediately upon admission?	• When does discharge planning start? 24 hours prior to discharge? Or within 24 hours of admit?
• How often are patients waiting in the ED/PACU for beds? How long do they wait? Overnight?	• Are there delays in ancillary (lab, radiology, etc.) test results?	• Are there issues with the timeliness of discharge, (e.g., 11 a.m.)?
• Does the organization "turn-away" patients due to ED diversion, cancelled surgeries, inability to accept transfers?	• Are there delays in bed cleaning and turnover? How are "ready" beds communicated?	• Are there opportunities to reduce LOS in key clinical areas?
• Is the current bed board automated or manual – how is it updated?	• Are there issues with timeliness, effectiveness or skills of transportation staff?	• Are there opportunities to reduce clinical denials? Technical denials?
• Does the organization use central scheduling with decision trees to facilitate appropriate placement?	• How efficient/productive is the OR suite? Are there delays in pre-admission testing, prep, PACU, etc.?	• Are there delays in post-acute placement for TCU, Rehab, Home Care, etc.?
• Who is accountable for determining if/when a bed is available? (Nursing, Admitting, Bed Control?)	• Are there delays in movement from ICUs to step-down or to general med/surg?	• Are patients often re-admitted for same or related diagnoses?

Note: ED, emergency department; PACU, post-anesthesia care unit; OR, operating room; ICU, intensive care unit; LOS, length of stay; TCU, transitional care unit.

FIGURE 8.7
Throughput Questions

Figure 8.8 shows the components of throughput as they relate to one another as a patient moves from admission to discharge. It may seem simplistic but is often a component of throughput that is left uncorrected, creating future issues that may eventually erode the work completed.

Figure 8.8 demonstrates an emphasis on discharge planning and execution across all areas. Due to the time required to access community services when needed, discharge planning should be a consideration as soon as a patient is admitted for treatment. One of the most important aspects of discharge planning is the education of the patient's family on the condition and extended care required. A family member or close friend helping with care will be more comfortable with his or her role if he or she has more than one chance to learn what he or she needs to be doing and what to watch out for. Reviewing throughput from the perspective of discharge is important from a financial standpoint as well. Hospitals may save more than $500 per day by ensuring patients do not stay longer than necessary.

Incorporating the three components of throughput shown in Figure 8.8 into a work plan allows managers to address each area with an interdisciplinary approach. The key work steps should engaging physicians in the process to apply standardized criteria for medical necessity, develop criteria for standardized admission and discharge, and create unit-specific admission and discharge criteria. Develop an

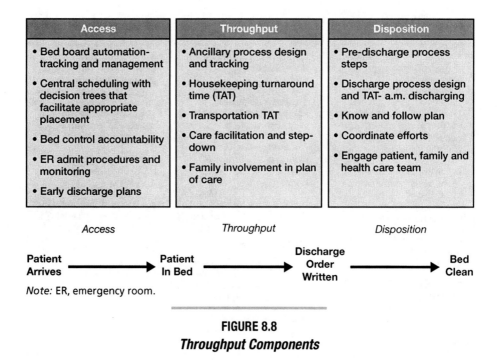

FIGURE 8.8
Throughput Components

oversight process to track compliance, outcomes, and allow enough flexibility for changes to be made when needed in an efficient time frame.

Operational Improvements Subgroup

The operational improvements subgroup is composed of case managers, nursing ancillary support staff, finance staff members, physicians, and analysts. This subgroup is responsible for the greatest amount of work, reviewing process maps prior to analysis, performing benchmark productivity tests for departments, and assessing patient flow. It is important that this subgroup be staffed with cooperative colleagues who bring insightful perspectives to the group, facilitating discussion without squabbling over smaller political matters within the hospital. If a patient were to be admitted to a hospital for open-heart surgery, for example, the state process map would be segmented into different episodes of care, beginning with early admission-based steps, continuing through the preparatory surgical steps, through the patient's movement, through various stages of care. Figure 8.9 provides greater detail for each step in a patient's individual throughput, demonstrating high-level steps through the preadmission process for surgical patients. Each segment of care is categorized by gaps in the process, shaded to match the category of gap with a list of the gaps.

The following process flow maps (Figures 8.10–8.12) further assess proper processes resulting from the work of the operational improvements group.

Once all new processes are in place, a final combined process map is created, approved, and tracked for compliance. Figure 8.13 would be an example of a final map, defining the processes, roles, and responsibilities for each task.

Overall clinical outcome data for patients in targeted DRGs, as well as those throughout an organization, should be made available to subgroups and should also detail infection rates, percentages of emergency room diversions, core measures, readmission rates, and adverse events.

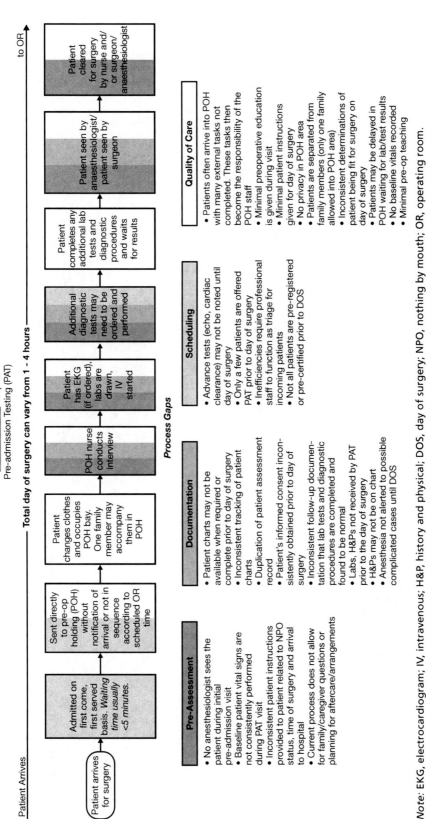

FIGURE 8.9

Current Pre-admission and DOS Process Flow

Note: EKG, electrocardiogram; IV, intravenous; H&P, history and physical; DOS, day of surgery; NPO, nothing by mouth; OR, operating room.

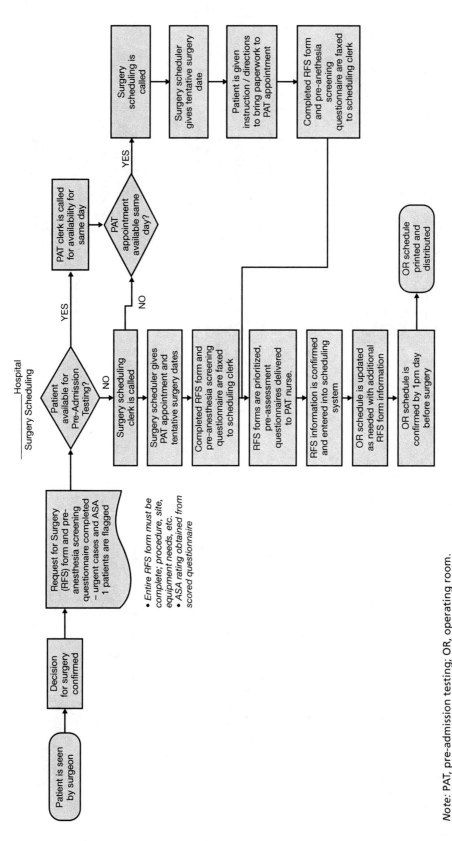

FIGURE 8.10
Future State Scheduling Process Flow

Note: PAT, pre-admission testing; OR, operating room.

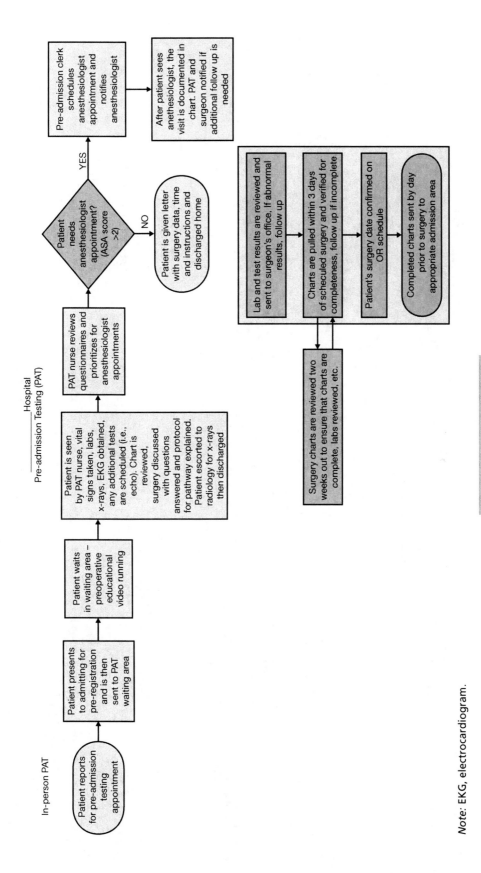

In-person PAT

Patient reports for pre-admission testing appointment

Patient presents to admitting for pre-registration and is then sent to PAT waiting area

Patient waits in waiting area – preoperative educational video running

Hospital
Pre-admission Testing (PAT)

Patient is seen by PAT nurse, vital signs taken, labs, x-rays, EKG obtained, any additional tests are scheduled (i.e., echo). Chart is reviewed, surgery discussed with questions answered and protocol for pathway explained. Patient escorted to radiology for x-rays then discharged

PAT nurse reviews questionnaires and prioritizes for anesthesiologist appointments

Patient needs anethesiologist appointment? (ASA score >2)

YES → Pre-admission clerk schedules anethesiologist appointment and notifies anesthesiologist

After patient sees anethesiologist, the visit is documented in chart. PAT and surgeon notified if additional follow up is needed

NO → Patient is given letter with surgery data, time and instructions and discharged home

Lab and test results are reviewed and sent to surgeon's office. If abnormal results, follow up

Charts are pulled within 3 days of scheculed surgery and verified for completeness, follow up if incomplete

Patient's surgery date confirmed on OR schedule

Completed charts sent by day prior to surgery to appropriate admission area

Surgery charts are reviewed two weeks out to ensure that charts are complete, labs reviewed, etc.

FIGURE 8.11
Future State PAT Process Flow

Note: EKG, electrocardiogram.

141

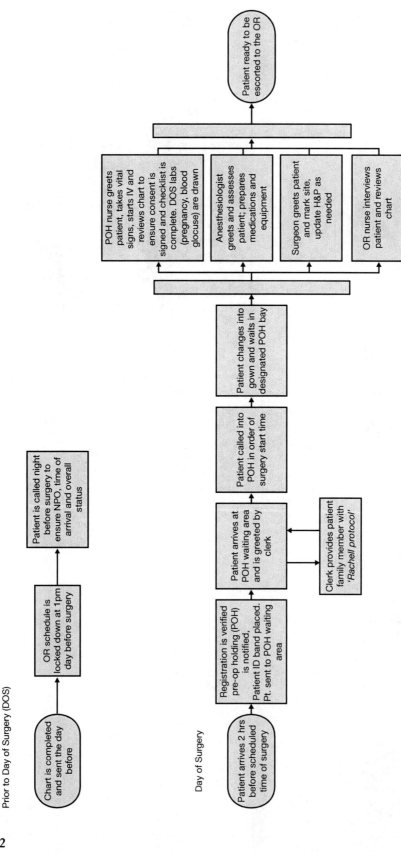

Prior to Day of Surgery (DOS)

Day of Surgery

——— Hospital

FIGURE 8.12

Future State Day of Surgery Process Flow

Note: OR, operating room; NPO, nothing by mouth; IV, intravenous; H&P, history and physical.

142

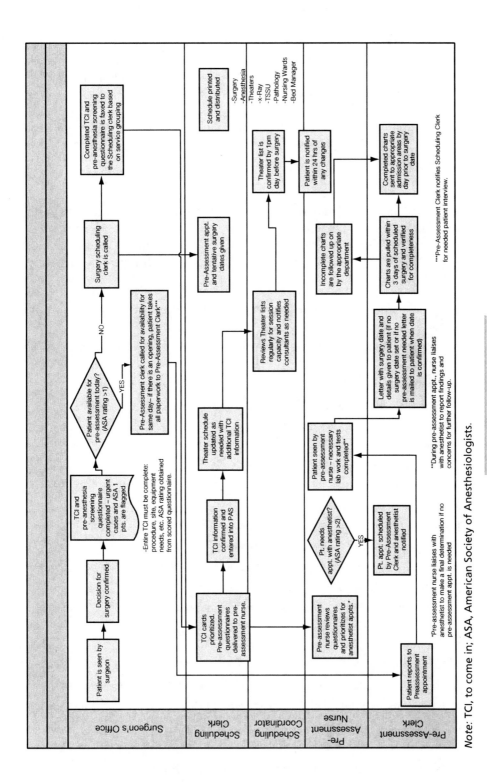

FIGURE 8.13

Future State Scheduling and Preassessment Process Flow

Note: TCI, to come in; ASA, American Society of Anesthesiologists.

143

Inviting Physicians

To identify which physicians should be invited into the operational improvements subgroup, identify physicians treating patients who exhibit greater LOS or costs per admission compared to benchmark figures, as well as physicians with numbers that adhere closer to a preferable median. Physicians with patients who fall into ranges that yield strong Medicare reimbursements are also prime candidates for inclusion because their resulting reimbursement income levels help keep hospitals solvent. Physicians with high patient infection rates or continued issues with quality outcomes should not be invited.

Data Collection

Once operational improvement subgroup team members are identified, and both processes and labor analyses are complete, it is time to align current labor and skill to appropriate episodes of care. An abundance of information should be made available to subgroups when comparing current versus future care pathways. The following hospital statistics are required:

- Hospital statistics for the prior fiscal or calendar year and for current year to date
  - Patient days and discharges—hospital, unit, ED, and operating room (OR) procedures
  - Average length of stay (ALOS), total and Medicare, and by unit
  - Average daily census (ADC) for hospital and by unit
  - Patient beds by nursing unit
  - Specialty by unit
  - Discharge by disposition by nursing unit
  - Denial data
- Number of days, discharges (cases), dollars (include downgrades, alternate level of care—e.g., subacute/skilled nursing facility (SNF)—observation)
- Reason codes for each category of denials
- Number of appeals (cases and number of days) and result in dollars
- Staffing levels for all related departments
  - Number of full-time equivalents (FTEs) by position, job titles, job descriptions, competencies
  - Staff assignments
- ED information
  - Number of visits in ED, diversion rate (and reason), use of observation status
  - Case management/social work staffing in ED
- OR statistics
  - Number of OR rooms
  - Number of beds in post-anesthesia care unit (PACU)
  - Back ups PACU to bed
  - OR delays and cancellations (by reason)

- Ancillary services
  - Reports on delays for lab reports, radiology reports, and cardiac caths
  - Electronic medical order sets for selected disease states
- Admission and discharge criteria by unit (particularly for specialty units—ICU, telemetry, step-down)
- Clinical utilization review criteria used
- Clinical pathways in use—different from the process maps the analysts will have created
- Description of case management/social service training/orientation program
- Copies of all forms or data collection tools used for case management/social services
- Department policies and procedures
- Additional data may be requested and collected during interviews and work observations

After reviewing statistical data, project analysts can begin to tie current state statistics to each episode of care process as mapped across the continuum of care by disease state and DRG. Special considerations should be taken into account when patients exhibit comorbidities, altering the framework in which their needs and pathways are assessed. Because each individual is different, flexibility needs to be built into the process within approved levels of variance, which will be identified as the new care pathways are developed.

The care pathways are created using the data at hand. Often, the current pathways may require little change. If they have been created with a multidisciplinary approach and are effective with analysis supporting, they are also cost effective. Current care pathways need to be segmented to match the episodes of care mapped by the analysts. This is often where one will find gaps in one's current care pathway, leading to undefined processes for documentation or transfer handoffs. The new care pathways need to be as detailed as possible. Although this may seem like expanding on the detail of the care, non-detailed pathways would create difficulty for staff to follow. The goal is to reduce variation, and once these elements are implemented, they actually reduce stress as each member of the care delivery team has a more defined responsibility.

Before labor and supplies are added to each step in the care pathway, the next step is to evaluate services provided at each step of the patient's care. This is where utilization of services becomes important. The variances of practice will be noted in this part of the workflow. The example used earlier where the orthopedic surgeon was not ambulating his patient until the second postoperative day, and then using an extra day of physical therapy, was discovered during this part of the work. Analysts may work with the education department or nursing team members to research standards of care, so both peer reviews and external studies can be evaluated before making final recommendations.

The final step in the development process occurs once care pathways are reviewed, created (or if preexisting, updated), both labor and supplies are mapped to appropriate segments, and those completion time lines are assigned to each episode of care. There are several resources available to develop final care pathways, as well as EBM order sets. Among them is the U.S. Department of Health and Human Services' Agency for Healthcare Research and Quality (http://www.ahrq.gov), which provides sample order sets based on listed conditions among other useful tools.

A partial example of a completed care pathway for a cardiac patient undergoing a coronary bypass graft is shown in Figure 8.14.

Once the care pathways are reviewed, created, or updated, labor and supplies are then mapped to each segment. Also, ensure that completion time lines are assigned for each episode of care.

Establishing Benchmark Reports

When analysts present cross-departmental labor benchmarking, the information provided will be a directional guide for focusing efforts, addressing variances, and quantifying productivity. The benchmarking report, however, is not intended to provide a set of recommendations for specific departmental changes because this requires further review of many additional components, such as skill sets, experience, acuity, or allocation of tasks within the labor force. A precise analysis of departmental work flows, bottlenecks, waste, or redundancy drills down into variances, allows for a more complete picture of labor needs. Team members must also realize that benchmarking is not a reflection of present or past management; it is merely a tool for analysis, adaptation, and progress.

After an initial assessment, subgroups should report findings to the multidisciplinary team. A review of services performed and utilization patterns should include resources allocated to other departments, to portray accurate departmental costs when multiple units work together during patient care. Each staffing change should quantify the financial impact of the change, including departmental recommendations and targets. In many cases, a shift in staff is more effective than eliminating staff because many nursing models call for the use of agency and temporary staff. After staffing allocations are reviewed, excess overtime costs should be reviewed for further savings.

Aligning Skills

Once labor benchmarking and correlating investigations into staffing needs are complete, skills should be aligned with episodes of care, representing the second step in the labor process. Incorporating the flex model (as described in Chapter 2) provides greater flexibility of task completion. By matching cases to nurse specialties, there is a greater opportunity to use all staff during routine cases. Staffing nurses based on patient needs can be repeated across the continuum of care for tasks, which do not require long spans of time. It is not intended to reduce the consistency of care for a patient with multiple handoffs, but rather it identifies areas where professional nurses are performing duties, which could be executed by support staff, better using advanced employees within a department.

Adding Time Lines

The next task given to the operational improvement subgroup is to assign expected clinical outcomes to each pathway. This task is accomplished by adding time lines for meeting core measures and by incorporating KPIs (infection rates, surgical case delays, turnaround times for lab results). The process should improve the quality of care with reduced costs, creating a baseline measurement of costs for reporting monthly KPIs and quality measures.

	Pre-op	Post-op	2 hrs	4 hrs	6 hrs	8 hrs	10 hrs	12 hrs
• Radiology	• CXR • Carotid US • Call surgeon with results	• CXR						
• Laboratory	• CBC, BMP, Mg, PT/PTT, BMBG, Type & Cross	• CBC, BMP, ABG, Mg, PT/PTT			• i-Stat (ABG, CBC, BMP, Mg)			
• Activity	• Ad lib • Activity level Assessment		• Turn ROM	• Turn ROM	• Turn ROM	• Recliner	• Bath	• Ambulate 25 feet
• Respiratory	• IS Instruction, ABG, Respiratory risk Assessment	• Wean vent		• Extubate	• IS Q 1 hr • CDB	• IS Q 1 hr • CDB	• IS Q 1 hr • CDB	• IS Q 1 hr • CDB
• Education	• PATTS/Pre-op instruction with patient and family	• Plan of care explained		• CDB, IS use • Increased activity • Pain control	→ (continues)			
• Diet	• NPO after midnight • Dietary risk assessment			• Sips/Chips	• Advanced diet as tolerated			
• Medications	• Obtain and document a complete list of pt's meds (TJC safety goal) • Consider beta blocker (recommended by the national voluntary consensus standards for cardiac surgery) • Prophylactic Antibiotic	• Pain meds PRN • Consider precedex • Administer hemodynamic drips as ordered • Glucose management			• Pain meds	→ (continues)		
• Treatments	• Actual weight							
• Family Support	• Pre-op instruction	• Consider family support • Plan of care explained • Keep updated • Consider clergy	→ (continues)					

FIGURE 8.14

Coronary Artery Bypass Graph Pathway

Note: CXR, chest X-ray; CBC, complete blood count; BMP, basic metabolic profile; PT/PTT, prothrombin time/partial thromboplastin time; BMBG, bedside monitoring blood glucose; ABG, arterial blood gas; ROM, range of motion; IS, inspiration spirometer; PATTS, pre-admission testing and teachings; NPO, nothing by mouth; CDB, chest deep breaths; PRN, as needed; TJC, The Joint Commission.

Surveying the Outcomes

Finally, this subgroup creates realistic surveys for each care pathway as they relate to physician, patient, and staff satisfaction. Quality outcomes will improve, costs will be reduced, and sustainability will be supported as participants realize the positive impacts and value of the resulting changes. Generic surveys for patients and staff are not taken seriously unless obvious issues exist; most surveys returned are unbalanced and generally negative. Specific surveys related to each pathway, however, allow for a more accurate reflection of perceived outcomes. Physicians will more likely respond to fewer questions if they are specific to areas which they deem important.

Supply Chain Process Subgroup

As the care pathway is aligned with labor, a similar process is performed with the type and quantity of supplies applied to each episode of care, which helps reduce costs through vendor consolidation and better item pricing. The key to this process is defining correct uses, range of amounts, and locations for product storage with consideration to care pathways. For more information on supply chain management, see Chapter 4.

The supply chain subgroup implements changes recommended by the operational improvements subgroup. Materials management, as described in Chapter 4, aims to keep costs under control while negotiating contracts and purchasing supplies. The challenge is keeping costs down when purchases are made outside of the department by individual doctors and units.

Product selection and expected volumes are determined through the care pathway process and the lists are then given the materials management. The contracting staff then review the options available to them and negotiate contracts that are presented to the team. Once vendors and products are approved, the contracts are finalized.

Contract management is also a task handled by this subgroup. The control of all contracts should be within the materials management department because independent buying and contracting by department managers allows multiple vendors into the system and erodes savings. Contracts executed by department managers who believe they have saved their department money with reduced costs may not realize the organization has other contracts that require levels of purchases. If one department displaces volume, the savings they obtained may negatively impact the pricing on all other departments.

The only way to prevent these occurrences is for a central repository and process. This does not preclude a department from requesting or bringing to the attention of the contracting staff vendors who offer discounts. It means contracting needs to be informed and leading the contracting process.

Although a complete product formulary cannot be created through the implementation of care pathways for a limited number of DRGs, a large amount of product categories can be standardized as we saw for linen, commodities, and intravenous (IV) supplies. The more important outcome is the communication and education of all staff and physicians that a product formulary with structured protocol for additions to the formulary is underway. Just like a drug formulary, materials management working with the value analysis team (VAT) should define the criteria for additions or substitutions to the formulary.

Treatment Subgroup

The treatment subgroup is responsible for developing tracking and reporting outcomes by using finance employees and analysts familiar with Six Sigma and LEAN principles. The addition of analysis training in these processes is becoming quite common even for small community hospitals. As a consultant, the problem of slippage or noncompliance recognized months later has always been a threat to project work. Working with clients and spending months on committee work only to find out later that old habits have returned or supply spending is increasing is as frustrating for the consultants as it is for the staff who worked hard to achieve changes that have not been sustained.

By following the processes outlined in this chapter, your department will become efficient and, more importantly, you will provide patient care with the correct skill sets and supplies for each segment of care. Safe and high-quality patient care can stay within budget as waste is removed and attention to the needs of each episode of care (EOC) is met.

9

Six Sigma

Nancy Bateman and Cynthia Tong

Becoming familiar with and using the Six Sigma approach to management will help you increase your budget while decreasing the amount of medical errors on your floor. This chapter introduces Six Sigma from its creation to the latest methodologies tailored to health care management. The five steps involved are introduced and then broken down to describe each element in its entirety. Using the Six Sigma tracking process will allow your department to thrive, along with utilizing the latest technologies in health care.

LEARNING OBJECTIVES

1. Be able to define Six Sigma.
2. List the five steps of Six Sigma.
3. Understand the value of using Six Sigma in health care.

SIX SIGMA AND ITS USE IN HEALTH CARE

Six Sigma is a management approach to quality improvement that was pioneered by Motorola and Toyota. Six Sigma optimizes operational processes and reduces inefficiencies by limiting procedural variations within an organization. The program has been adopted in health care, and has helped organizations contain cost increases and reduce medical errors.

In 1998, Commonwealth Health Corporation (CHC) was the first organization to introduce Six Sigma to health care. CHC is a 500-bed multisite system with headquarters in Bowling Green, Kentucky. The corporation's $900,000 investment in Six Sigma resulted in throughput improvements in their radiology department, reducing costs per procedure within the department. This led to a savings of more than $2.5 million for CHC and a 2.8:1 return on investment (van den Heuvel, Does, & Verver, 2005).

Another example of a hospital achieving outstanding results with Six Sigma can be found in the Red Cross Hospital, a 384-bed general hospital in Beverwijk, the Netherlands. Through the seven projects that were initiated, the Red Cross Hospital experienced the following:

1. A shortening in the length of stay of chronic obstructive pulmonary disease (COPD) patients
2. A reduction of errors in invoices from temporary agencies
3. A revision of terms of payment of their supplier contracts
4. A reduction in the number of mistakes on patient invoices
5. A reduction in the number of patients on intravenous antibiotics (van den Heuvel, Does, & Bisgard, 2005).

Although these changes appear modest individually, their overall effect had a significant impact on the hospital. Each of the successes was obtained through a small change or adjustment in their operations, but these minor changes helped the hospital better manage their patients. The successful implementation of Six Sigma has since been documented to help many other health care organizations and remains a popular approach to achieving organization-wide quality improvement processes.

Six Sigma projects are typically led by Master Black Belts (MBBs) or Black Belts (BBs) and include Yellow Belts (YBs) and/or Green Belts (GBs). These designations signify certain accreditation levels within the Six Sigma program, functioning similarly to, and based on the naming construct levels of knowledge within, martial arts training.

The origins of Six Sigma are based on scientific principles that aim to achieve no more than 3.4 defective parts per million (dppm) within a manufacturing operation. Within nonmanufacturing organizations, Six Sigma provides a project management structure that seeks streamlined decision making. The project management structure is defined by the acronym DMAIC (Define, Measure, Analyze, Improve, and Control). DMAIC is a process that eliminates operational inefficiencies or waste (known as MUDA—a Japanese term for wasteful activity) by applying systematic improvement. The five phases of Six Sigma are listed in Table 9.1.

Executing the structure of DMAIC in any organization requires time and expense, so a cost-effectiveness analysis should be performed before any projects begin, ensuring that the efficiency gains outweigh the implementation costs. Two indicators that a project requires DMAIC are that the problem is complex and that the risks of the solutions are high. For any Six Sigma project to succeed, it is important to not skip any of the DMAIC steps.

■ **Define**—The first step of any Six Sigma project is to Define objectives and gain consensus among team members and support from executive sponsors. This step should be completed within two weeks. If the process takes longer, it could be a sign that the scope of the project is too broad or too vague. If this is the case, it is advisable to meet with sponsors and re-scope the project. Key steps in Define are as follows:
1. Draft and review a project charter.
2. Validate the problem and goals by reviewing existing data. In order to proceed, the problem identified must (a) exist, (b) be important to the

TABLE 9.1
Five Steps of Six Sigma

Define	Identify the problem
	Set requirements and goals
	Validate voice of the customer (VOC)
Measure	Value stream map/process flow
	Measure process
	Collect baseline data
Analyze	Validate hypothesis
	Identify root cause of problem
	Prioritize root causes
Improve	Develop possible solutions
	Test solutions
	Measure results and standardize solutions
Control	Develop training plan
	Implement solution/new streamlined process
	Continue to monitor and measure

Note: Adapted from Pande, P. S., Neuman, R. P., & Cavanagh, R. R. (2002). *The Six Sigma way team fieldbook: An implementation guide for process improvement teams.* New York, NY: McGraw-Hill.

customer, (c) be important to the business, and (d) reasonably be achieved through the Six Sigma process.

3. Validate benefits by estimating the financial impact of the project.
4. Validate the scope of the project.
5. Develop a communication plan.
6. Draft a work plan (including budgeting, milestones, timeline).

▪ **Measure**—The objective of Measure is to understand current problems by collecting and reviewing data. During this process, teams determine the processes that will be used to affect positive changes. Baseline measurements should be considered in this step, and definitions of improvement goals should be refined. The key elements in Measure are as follows:

1. Develop a value stream map to understand the current process flow.
2. Identify the inputs, outputs, and any variables related to the current process.
3. Develop a plan for collecting data.
4. Determine how the data will be analyzed.
5. Start collecting data to establish a baseline.

▪ **Analyze**—The purpose of Analyze is to pinpoint the root cause of problems during critical points in the decision-making process. As the previous step was critical in collecting reliable data, this step is equally important in being critical about the data collection process. Key steps to Analyze are as follows:

1. Analyze the process flow to identify the cause and effect.
2. Identify a benchmark to track improvements gained through the process change.

3. Analyze the data collected in Measure.

4. Prioritize by using tools like a Pareto diagram. *Pareto diagrams* focus on the most critical items for consideration and improvement, based on the principle that 20% of issues create 80% of problems within a system.

5. Collect any additional data needed.

■ **Improve**—By the Improve step, initial hypotheses have either been validated or dispelled. At this stage, the scope of a project should be defined resolutely, and pilot tests should be executed before the full implementation of new policies. The following steps are essential for Improve to be successful:

1. Develop, evaluate, and select potential solutions.

2. Create the new value stream map, which designs material flow to bring services to consumers.

3. Pilot testing

4. Collect data as defined in Measure, comparing to the baseline for improvement measurement.

5. Execute full implementation plan.

■ **Control**—Control is a sign of project completion; solutions should be tested and ready for use. The transition plan should uphold the expectation of maintaining the gains achieved. The transition plans should be easy to follow for process participants and should ensure that the new models are executed properly. Remember to work out any kinks prior to transition. Key steps for Control are as follows:

1. Develop a standard operating procedure, ensuring that the new process is sustained by owners and lessens the risk of variability.

2. Monitor fully executed implementation, collecting and measuring data throughout the life of the process.

3. Validate performance by measuring cost savings or new revenue.

4. Complete the project.

APPLYING SIX SIGMA TO IMPROVING HEALTH CARE OUTCOMES

Proper use of Six Sigma will result in better operational efficiency, higher process quality, and cost effectiveness. Potential problem areas should be identified within the three basic quality-of-care categories: overuse, underuse, and misuse. Not addressing and revising these problems will cost the health care industry billions of dollars a year. Using Six Sigma to design and refine patient care processes eliminates the need to retrace steps, correct reporting errors, redo examinations, or reschedule appointments. Although there have already been statistical tools to measure and improve quality such as Total Quality Management (TQM) and Continuous Quality Improvement (CQI), Six Sigma produces the best results. Factors accounting for its success include:

■ The instillation of a common language and shared techniques

■ A rigorous control mechanism is provided, and adherence is required

- Leadership support is driven by those most involved in the process
- Variability process is targeted, rather than aiming at averages
- Organizational vision is aligned and supported

The first steps in Six Sigma reduce process variation, instituting practices that create standard lengths and procedures within instances of patient care. Evaluate entire projects and break them down into their composing parts, making the progress more organized and less overwhelming. After segments are clearly defined, project goals, scoping finds, anticipated solutions, and results should be measured (Van Kooy & Pexton, 2005).

The following scenario details common steps within a Six Sigma project. In this example, executive sponsors briefed teams with the following details:

- The hospital is continually being challenged to reduce waits and delays for patients coming into inpatient beds.
- Inpatient bed demand exceeds current capacity, and a significant variation in bed assignment within the hospital has contributed to delays.
- Increasing bed capacity is not an option and will not solve process flow problems.
- Placing patients in correct units to receive proper levels of care provides an impact on safety and finance.
- An efficient bed assignment process is one of the core processes for a hospital.
- Hospital administration realizes the need to optimize access and improve overall satisfaction.

Table 9.2 illustrates a sample project. Charter teams composed of stakeholders and process owners are led by a Master Black Belt and a Black Belt.

Having defined problem statements and project goals, there is a clear understanding of expected outcomes. The next steps seek to build consensus and agreement among team members and stakeholders, identifying customers, and developing a high-level work plan. In many cases, customers will be the process owners, team members, and external customers.

The Measure step comprised collecting data, processing value stream maps, and establishing baseline measures. A value stream map (Figure 9.1) helps teams understand current bed assignment processes.

During this phase, it is helpful to get input from several process owners, usually uncovering that there are several "right" procedures and many variables involved in current processes. In this example, there are redundant steps that can be eliminated after teams start measuring sample data points to develop a baseline of productivity. Because the objective of this project is to reduce turnover time from admit orders to bed assignment to 15 minutes, the current baseline turnaround time should be established using data from emergency department (ED) and post-anesthesia care unit (PACU). This can be accomplished by reviewing patient charts or by manually logging bed assignment time.

With data in tow, the project can move forward to the Analyze phase. The value stream mapping of the current process creates outlines that demonstrate how we can outline strengths and weaknesses in current processes.

TABLE 9.2
Project Charter

Problem Statement	Team
The inefficient bed assignment process increases patient length of stay time in ED holding area, physician's office, or PACU.	Unit clerks Administrative coordinator/house supervisor Registration/admitting Charge nurse Admitting physician (high-volume admits) Case manager IS analyst/network
	Coach
	Master Black Belt Black Belt
Goal/Objective	**Deliverables (potential)**
To decrease patient bed assignment process for patients admitted for a total improved turnover time of 15 minutes from time of request.	1. Develop a streamlined process for bed assignment. 2. Reduce bed assignment time to 15 minutes from request for admission to bed assigned. 3. Develop a dashboard to continually monitor compliance of new time benchmark.

Note: ED, emergency department; PACU, post-anesthesia care unit; IS, information systems.

Strengths

■ There are sufficient personnel staffed to accomplish the initiative.

■ Good relationships with physicians exist to monitor the voice of the customer (VOC).

■ Excellent working relationships exist within the departments.

■ There is buy-in and support from senior administration and department leaders.

Weaknesses

■ There is no consistency in the current process; it is very dependent on staff personnel and causes challenges during shift changes.

■ Not one department or person is responsible 24–7 for the bed assignment process, which adds to the variability experienced.

■ There is a lack of consistent communication style and/or tools (i.e., beeper, telephone, and computer) within departments (nursing unit, housekeeping, and transport).

■ No regularly scheduled bed management meetings exist.

With this information, leaders can create a fishbone diagram (illustrated in Figure 9.2). The diagram is typically used in Six Sigma projects to help identify bottlenecks, weaknesses, and constraints within a current process.

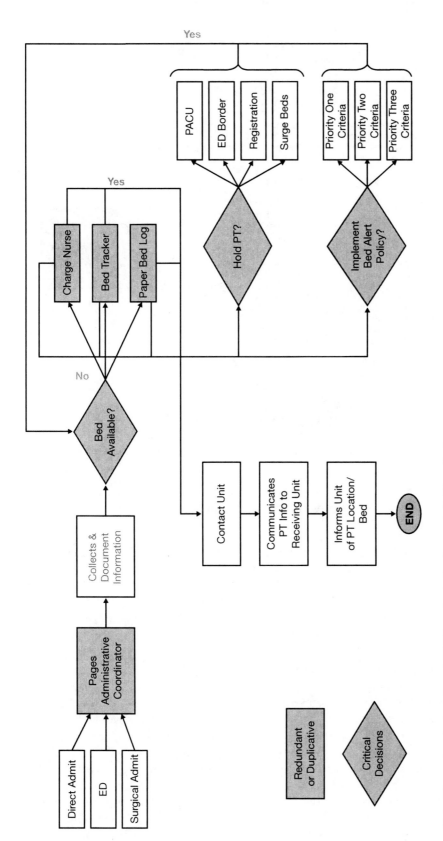

FIGURE 9.1
Current State Bed Assignment Process Flow

Note: ED, emergency department; PACU, post-anesthesia care unit; PT, patient.

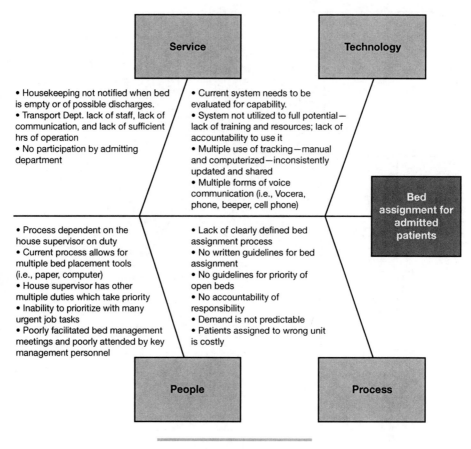

FIGURE 9.2
Process Breakdown Fishbone

A sample Pareto diagram for the bed placement processes is shown in Figure 9.3, helping to identify cycles and accounting problems within processes.

In the example shown in Figure 9.3, it was discovered that the bed assignment cycle was the root of the problem. Developing and gathering the data shown earlier can take anywhere from one week to one month, depending on current systems and available information. It is important to analyze data thoroughly, because it is essential to a well-defined decision-making process. With every element of bed assignment measured and analyzed, brainstorming for solutions can begin. Taking the existing process flow as a guide, teams can create a "new-state" process flow map, allowing for all solutions to be visually represented. The illustration shown in Figure 9.4 is an example of the new proposed process for bed assignment of admitted patients.

The next step in the process calls for a pilot program to test revised turnaround times. After drafting the new streamlined process, train pilot participants to check for potential complications. After achieving and documenting success with a pilot program, finalize the new procedures by delivering the plan to process owners. A tracking mechanism should be developed in order to maintain and measure the gains; some metrics for measuring bed assignment are illustrated in Table 9.3. Along with the dashboard, tracking sources for all data elements should be documented.

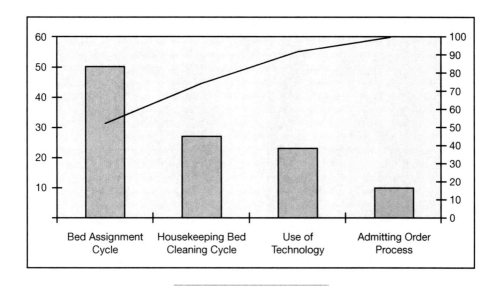

FIGURE 9.3
Bed Assignment Metrics

SUMMARY

As health care costs increase along with uncompensated care, health care leaders are faced with the tough decisions of cutting costs and eliminating waste. If an organization invests in minor operational adjustments, their impacts can be very large.

Listed in the following text are the expected areas that will benefit from a resource management project. Using the process and training subgroups allow these standards to be repeated for different diagnosis-related groups (DRGs), and each new DRG will be established in increasingly shorter timeframes. Each DRG processed through the newly structured system will have increasing overlap and fewer substructures to tackle. Areas listed afterward will require less adaptation as only minor DRG-specific changes will be needed.

- **Case management**—Review of models, staffing levels, and schedules will overlap.
- **Bed placement and management**—Establishment of these processes occur earlier in the process.
- **Scheduling process**—For surgical, diagnostic, and interventional studies, added DRG staffing will be addressed as necessary.
- **Admission criteria**—Consensus on vendor use or admission protocol.
- **Communication**—A model is created at the beginning of any project and should continue as planned throughout an organization.
- **Staffing**—Staffing levels and skills to match each EOC will be different for each DRG, but the staff determining these levels will remain consistent.
- **Training and job function changes**—Training and job function responsibilities will be similar for grouped DRGs.

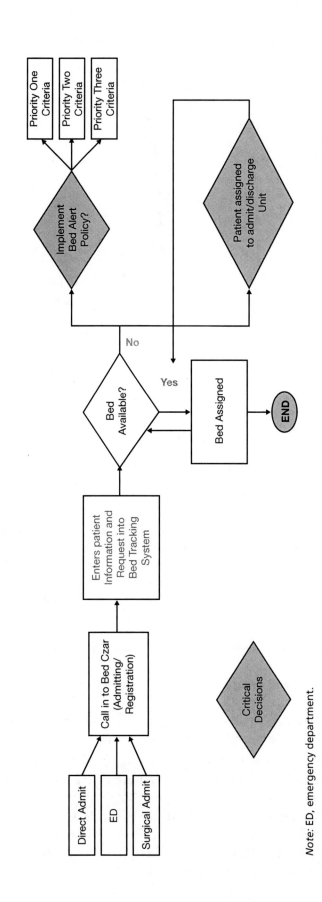

FIGURE 9.4
Proposed "New" Bed Assignment Process Flow

Note: ED, emergency department.

TABLE 9.3
Bed Assignment Dashboard

	Time/Minutes
Bed request input into Star System	1 Minutes
Review vacant beds on unit	1-3 Minutes
Verify with charge nurse appropriate	3-5 Minutes
Assign bed	1 Minutes
Communicate bed assignment to unit	3 Minutes
Update Star System	1 Minutes
Total Bed Assignment Procedure Time	≤ 15 Minutes

	Tracking Source
Bed request input into Star System	Star
Review vacant beds on unit	Star
Verify with charge nurse appropriate	Star
Assign bed	Star
Communicate bed assignment to unit	Beeper Computer Log System
Update Star System	Star

- **Policy and procedure changes**—It is important to keep policy changes consistent across applications to new and existing DRGs.

- **Any facility or space constraints**—Consideration of facility and space constraints should be included in the review of new policy and process changes.

Along with the previous checklist items and overlapping DRG processing improvements, the list that follows demonstrates the final steps before implementing final recommendations for improvement.

- **Timing and sequencing of the action steps**—Anytime multiple changes are necessary, it is critical to determine which changes occur first and establish a work plan for introducing each step. Make sure the organizational culture allows enough time to complete each change. If parallel changes are occurring, also include milestones for each step to track each progress point.

- **List of any equipment or capital costs associated with recommended changes**—During the process, executive team members will want to know the return on investment (ROI) of the change processes. When calculating the savings or improved revenue, remember to account for costs and equipment needed.

With any effort taken to achieve change, improvements must be tracked adequately for sustainability. This can be done by establishing targeted goals and outcomes and by making improvements against baseline averages. Tracked line-item improvements are called key performance indicators (KPIs) and should be included

TABLE 9.4

Monthly Key Performance Indicators

Key Performance Indicator	Baseline	Target or Budget Variance	Feb-10	Mar-10	Apr-10	May-10	Jun-10	Jul-10	Aug-10
Financials									
Revenue									
Salaries and Wages									
Overtime									
Medical Supplies									
Other Supplies/Purchased Services									
Other Expenses									
Rent & Education									
Repairs and Maintenance									
Total Expenses									
Statistics									
Average Daily Census									
Average Length of Stay									
Total Patient Days									
A & E Visits									
Outpatient Visits									
Inpatient Surgeries									
Day Surgeries									
Quality/Service/People									
Infection Rate									
Mortality - # of Deaths									
Patient Satisfaction Score									
Staff Satisfaction Score									
Turnover rate									
% LWOB									
ED Wait Times									
% of ED Diverts									
Supply Chain									
Total Supply Spend per Adjusted Patient Days									
Supply Cost per OR case									
Supply Cost per Cath Lab									
Surgery									
Overall Utilization									
% On Time Starts									
% Cancellations									
% Overtime									
CMI	Indicators								

Note: A&E, accident and emergency; LWOB, left without being seen; ED, emergency departmenrt; OR, operating room.

in a dashboard so all improvements are viewed monthly in one report. The dashboard should show baselines, targeted goals, and each month's results. Many overlapping improvements can backslide if not maintained, making KPI grouping essential. Some of the KPIs often tracked in resource management projects, depending on the DRGs under review, are as follows:

- Targeted increased revenue in the ED
- Targeted savings for decreased LOS
- Targeted increased patient, staff, and physician satisfaction against baseline
- Targeted percentage of reduced delays and cancellations in the operating room (OR), catheterization laboratory and patient appointment wait times
- Targeted reduction for LWBS (left without being seen) in the ED with reduced divert status

Table 9.4 is a dashboard template that can be adjusted as needed. It is important to limit KPIs because adding too many will lessen the impact of reports. Dashboards should be a one-page read because the executive team and research method subgroups will not take the time to review monthly results.

Using the Six Sigma methodology will aid you in perfecting the management of your resources. These advancements will increase your budget while providing higher quality of care. By outlining the five steps of Six Sigma and breaking them down for a more detailed description, any part of the process should be easy to reference when needed.

Conclusion

Nancy Bateman and Jacklyn Mead

CASE STUDY

This case study highlights segments of a project in which top diagnosis-related groups (DRGs) were identified by length-of-stay issues. The hospital in this case study also had system-wide issues with overtime and denials related to use of observation status. Goals of the project were to improve throughput, reduce overtime, and restrict use of observation days. This hospital's project eventually evolved into developing DRG-specific pathways, but administrators wanted to improve system-wide issues first.

The first step in the project was data collection and analysis of top DRGs for costs and lengths of stay. The results of the top 15 DRGs are shown in Table IV.1. The table represents the Medicare severity-diagnosis-related group (MS-DRG) opportunity days based on case-rate-only payers (5,195 discharges or 45.6% of all discharges). The total cost savings opportunity based on a $400 variable cost per day is $836,654, representing 39.5% of all discharges and 7.9% of patient days.

Table IV.2 reports the opportunity for the same top 15 MS-DRGs, with outliers representing 13.6% of the total outlier population. Certain conditions of extended length of stay or cost of care above the thresholds set by the Centers for Medicare and Medicaid Services (CMS) for that year may be submitted for increased reimbursements. However, reducing the number of outliers is a cost savings because reimbursement for outliers do not guarantee coverage of all costs of care. Table IV.2 shows a savings opportunity of $631,539 based on a $400 variable cost per day. The target is to reduce outlier patient days by 10% through improved care coordination and throughput.

The next step is to determine which patients were responsible for the greatest number of outlier days. Table IV.3 shows that outlier populations were concentrated by more than 50% in respiratory and circulatory clinical diagnoses. This is not surprising, because it is common to see issues in these major diagnostic categories (MDCs). Usually, the cause is lack of availability of long-term-care beds in the community.

The next issue addressed was the high percentage of observation admits. When patients arrive at a hospital and it is unclear if they should be admitted or discharged, they can be admitted under the observation status.

In the case of this hospital, an abnormal amount of patients were admitted as observation patients, because case managers that were assigned to the emergency department (ED) were only there from 10:00 a.m. to 10:00 p.m. and were the sole

TABLE IV.1
Top 15 MS-DRGs With Opportunity

MS-DRG	MS-DRG Title	A Cases	B Tomball ALOS	C CMS GLOS	D CMS Truncated LOS	A*(B-D) Opportunity Days	Opportunity $
690	KIDNEY & URINARY TRACT INFECTIONS W/O MCC	171	5.06	3.50	3.79	216.8	$ 86,702
193	SIMPLE PNEUMONIA & PLEURISY W MCC	174	7.14	5.30	6.10	181.8	72,737
689	KIDNEY & URINARY TRACT INFECTIONS W MCC	102	6.82	4.80	5.41	144.2	57,680
190	CHRONIC OBSTRUCTIVE PULMONARY DISEASE W MCC	107	6.05	4.70	5.28	82.5	33,017
291	HEART FAILURE & SHOCK W MCC	146	6.26	5.00	5.71	80.4	32,159
603	CELLULITIS W/O MCC	123	4.83	3.80	4.25	70.7	28,288
280	ACUTE MYOCARDIAL INFARCTION, DISCHARGED ALIVE W MCC	34	8.03	5.40	6.10	65.7	26,267
300	PERIPHERAL VASCULAR DISORDERS W CC	33	6.82	4.00	5.05	58.5	23,395
872	SEPTICEMIA OR SEVERE SEPSIS W/O MV 96+ HOURS W/O MCC	67	5.73	4.60	4.95	52.2	20,886
191	CHRONIC OBSTRUCTIVE PULMONARY DISEASE W CC	35	5.83	4.00	4.42	49.3	19,719
194	SIMPLE PNEUMONIA & PLEURISY W CC	65	5.34	4.30	4.61	47.0	18,815
863	POSTOPERATIVE & POST-TRAUMATIC INFECTIONS W/O MCC	20	7.15	4.10	4.88	45.4	18,162
377	G.I. HEMORRHAGE W MCC	39	6.62	4.90	5.50	43.6	17,450
248	PERC CARDIOVASC PROC W NON-DRUG-ELUTING STENT W MCC OR 4+ VES/STENTS	23	7.09	4.30	5.28	41.6	16,623
	All Others	913				911.9	364,751
		2,052				2,091.6	$ 836,654

Note: MS-DRG, Medicare severity-diagnosis-related group; ALOS, average length of stay; CMS, Centers for Medicare and Medicaid; GLOS, geometric mean length of stay; MCC, major complications and comorbidities; CC, complications and comorbidities; MV, mechanical ventilation; GI, gastrointestinal; LOS, length of stay.

TABLE IV.2

Savings Through Reduced Outliers

MS-DRG	MS-DRG Title	A Cases	B Tomball ALOS	C CMS GLOS	D CMS Truncated LOS	A*(B-D) Opportunity Days	Opportunity $
291	HEART FAILURE & SHOCK W MCC	7	25.4	5.0	5.7	138.0	$ 55,213
603	CELLULITIS W/O MCC	6	22.0	3.8	4.3	106.5	42,590
193	SIMPLE PNEUMONIA & PLEURISY W MCC	4	29.0	5.3	6.1	91.6	36,642
189	PULMONARY EDEMA & RESPIRATORY FAILURE	6	20.5	4.7	6.4	84.9	33,948
690	KIDNEY & URINARY TRACT INFECTIONS W/O MCC	6	15.3	3.5	3.8	69.3	27,702
689	KIDNEY & URINARY TRACT INFECTIONS W MCC	3	28.3	4.8	5.4	68.8	27,508
176	PULMONARY EMBOLISM W/O MCC	2	33.0	4.3	4.7	56.5	22,617
602	CELLULITIS W MCC	2	31.5	5.5	6.6	49.9	19,959
300	PERIPHERAL VASCULAR DISORDERS W CC	2	29.5	4.0	5.0	48.9	19,563
280	ACUTE MYOCARDIAL INFARCTION, DISCHARGED ALIVE W MCC	1	47.0	5.4	6.1	40.9	16,361
393	OTHER DIGESTIVE SYSTEM DIAGNOSES W MCC	1	45.0	4.9	6.3	38.7	15,484
252	OTHER VASCULAR PROCEDURES W MCC	1	45.0	5.3	7.1	37.9	15,154
593	SKIN ULCERS W CC	1	46.0	4.9	9.3	36.7	14,663
292	HEART FAILURE & SHOCK W CC	3	16.0	3.9	4.3	35.2	14,081
871	SEPTICEMIA OR SEVERE SEPSIS W/O MV 96+ HOURS W MCC	2	24.0	5.4	6.8	34.4	13,776
	All Other DRGs	48				640.7	256,278
		95				1,578.8	$ 631,539

Note: MS-DRG, Medicare severity-diagnosis-related group; ALOS, average length of stay; CMS, Centers for Medicare and Medicaid; GLOS, geometric mean length of stay; MCC, major complications and comorbidities; CC, complications and comorbidities; LOS, length of stay; MV, mechanical ventilation; DRGs, diagnosis-related groups.

TABLE IV.3

Concentration of Outliers

MDC	MDC Title	Cases	Opportunity Days	Opportunity $
05	DISEASES & DISORDERS OF THE CIRCULATORY SYSTEM	30	482.5	$ 193,004
04	DISEASES & DISORDERS OF THE RESPIRATORY SYSTEM	18	354.5	141,798
09	DISEASES & DISORDERS OF THE SKIN, SUBCUTANEOUS TISSUE & BREAST	10	211.2	84,488
11	DISEASES & DISORDERS OF THE KIDNEY & URINARY TRACT	9	138.0	55,210
08	DISEASES & DISORDERS OF THE MUSCULOSKELETAL SYSTEM & CONN TISSUE	4	77.4	30,955
18	INFECTIOUS & PARASITIC DISEASES, SYSTEMIC OR UNSPECIFIED SITES	5	76.7	30,662
01	DISEASES & DISORDERS OF THE NERVOUS SYSTEM	6	70.3	28,108
06	DISEASES & DISORDERS OF THE DIGESTIVE SYSTEM	3	56.5	22,584
23	FACTORS INFLUENCING HLTH STAT & OTHR CONTACTS WITH HLTH SERVCS	3	38.5	15,435
10	ENDOCRINE, NUTRITIONAL & METABOLIC DISEASES & DISORDERS	2	28.2	11,293
07	DISEASES & DISORDERS OF THE HEPATOBILIARY SYSTEM & PANCREAS	2	22.8	9,116
16	DISEASES & DISORDERS OF BLOOD, BLOOD FORMING ORGANS, IMMUNOLOG DISORD	2	17.6	7,041
21	INJURIES, POISONINGS & TOXIC EFFECTS OF DRUGS	1	4.6	1,844
		95	1578.8	$ 631,539

Note: MDC, major diagnostic categories.

168

providers of initial patient evaluations. Case managers did not participate or engage in discharge planning for patients, and rather than take the risk of discharging patients without adequate planning, they admitted patients to improve ED through-put or gave patients observation status. This helped the ED but created a negative impact to the nursing floors. In this case, improving the management of patient observation and converting them to inpatients when required would increase revenue as inpatients are reimbursed higher than observation patients. When observation patients end up staying more than 24 hours before being converted to more appropriate statuses, revenue is lost. This is shown in Table IV.4.

Through observations, interviews, and analysis, several contributing factors were identified for the excessive length of stays and increasing use of observation status. With case managers in the ED only conducting initial reviews, patients were handed over to ED physicians to make care decisions. ED physicians were then dealing with multiple levels of patient conditions. To move questionable patients through the ED process, observation status was applied because it provided a chance for monitoring symptoms without the risk of early discharge. A second possible cause was a lack of sufficient long-term-care beds in the hospital. Observation status allowed patients to receive care while waiting for beds to become available. Medical necessity may not indicate an inpatient stay, but without lower-level care available, the hospital was left with fewer options for patient placement.

Another issue identified was the requirement of consulting physicians to assess patients within 24 hours. Short-stay conditions alone could delay discharge by up to a day depending on admission timing. Patients were treated by attending physicians, with no medical director to oversee a clinical decision unit, therefore patient stays were dependent on each physician's timing of rounds. Additionally, clinical documentation by attending physicians was often vague, which did not provide enough information for care managers on the floors to support patient progression and discharge planning.

The hospital's case management model used a three-team approach, including a registered nurse (RN), a social worker, and a registered nurse acting as a utilization manager. There was no clerical support to the case management program, and communication between the two RNs and the patient's physician were not always coordinated. The social worker focused on patient family counseling and did not support discharge needs. Nothing in the program focused on reducing readmissions, and patients were only evaluated two to three times a week.

This hospital opted to tackle the systemic issues before beginning work on isolated DRGs. Once case management updated their model and added support for

TABLE IV.4
Observation Usage

	Conservative	Mid Range	Aggressive
Benchmark: Observation %	22%	20%	18%
Observation status patients converted	452	657	862
Potential Net IP Revenue (based on $3,500 per patient conversion)	$ 1,583,680	$ 2,300,550	$ 3,017,420

Note: IP, inpatient.

managing more patients, they were ready to work on pathways specific to the selected DRGs. Steps taken to advance the case management program included revising the current case management model to become more proactive, changing the focus to become patient centric and provide facilitation across the care continuum, and job descriptions were rewritten with clearly defined expectations, case-manager-to-patient ratios were established at 1:20, and social worker ratios were also set to 1:40. No ratios had been established within the prior model, and patient reviews were not tracked. Additionally, a physician advisor role was approved and filled.

The expectation in the new model is that case managers will perform a review of patients and communicate with nursing staff daily. The responsibilities of the program also allow case managers to support facilitation of care by clarifying treatment plans as necessary and removing barriers to care delivery. In this example, case managers were held accountable for measurable patient outcomes and communication between all care providers.

A clerical support position was also filled. Besides helping with communication and reporting, the clerical staff was able to call in for routine insurance updates and utilization reviews.

Once improvements were implemented, the hospital saw reduced length of stays, improved reimbursements (fewer days were denied because of lack of documentation), improved patient and physician satisfaction, and improved patient safety statistics.

A full-time case manager position was assigned to the ED 7 days a week. Responsibilities included documenting and supporting decisions that assisted with reducing the use of observation status. Additionally, the improvements in case management and throughput could not have been as successful had the physicians not engaged.

Table IV.5 matches improvements to physician involvement.

TABLE IV.5
Improvements Tied to Physician Involvement

Care Management	Physician Involvement
Daily "huddles" between nursing, care management staff and hospitalists of physician advisors	Reliable use of order sets, guidelines and protocols, where available
Seven day a week in house staffing	Physician-to-physician communication for consults
Extended hour staffing (12 hours a day versus 8 hours a day)	Prompt response to consult requests, as required to provide effective, efficient care, and avoid delays
ED case manager role	Early morning discharge orders
All elective surgical and procedural patients are reviewed for appropriate patient status (IP/OP) to procedure (to ensure precertification is in place)	Prompt response to ED and floors, and prompt visit if requesting that patient be held for physician to see
Twice daily review of all observation cases; all cases requiring change from inpatient to observation require secondary review	Daily collaboration with Case Managers and Physician Advisor(s)
Weekly problem solving and plan setting for long LOS patients	Ownership of patients when covering for colleagues; complete sign-outs, willingness of covering physicians to make treatment and disposition decisions on weekends/holidays.
Daily and weekly reports (dependent on available technology) to drive or re-align staffing priorities	Daily clinical goal setting, collaboratively with the care team and communicated to the patient, with pre-planning of discharges

Note: ED, emergency department; IP, inpatient; OP, outpatient; LOS, length of stay.

Once system issues were improved, the project changed its focus to review original DRGs. The following were chosen by the hospital:

- **Septicemia**—The hospital wanted to improve the ability for early identification and rapid testing. They also desired more aggressive management of the patients with automatic triggers for specialty consultants and engagement of pharmacy.
- **Congestive heart failure**—Was chosen to implement programs to identify high risk patients, incorporate education programs and outreach programs, and reduce length of stay and supply costs.
- **Bariatrics**—The hospital had scheduled the launch of a bariatric program and wanted care pathways and order sets developed. Because capital equipment purchases would be needed, requests and supply costs were evaluated. Targeted costs per case were established so program costs and service line profitability could be tracked.
- **Total hip and knee replacements**—An obvious choice because this DRG has less variation in the delivery care model, and rewards on supply costs and lengths of stay can be substantial.

Process maps for patient care flow were developed and tied to staffing and supplies. As mentioned earlier, a full productivity assessment was performed across the system because many departments are used for these DRGs. Full productivity benchmarking revealed a cost savings opportunity of $10 to $15 million across the system. A summary of the analysis is demonstrated in Table IV.6.

Nonlabor assessments identified a total of $2 to $6 million, with $278,000 to $786,000 identified in savings for total hip and knee implants. Further analysis reviewed commodities, surgical packs, and other supporting supplies used for both total joints as well as bariatric supplies. A complete listing of the initiatives with savings identified is listed in Table IV.7.

Once all supplies are reviewed, and both productivity and process maps are completed, the last step is to create care pathways and order sets. Each episode of care (EOC) was identified with staffing levels, required skill sets, and standardized supplies and services. When the project was completed, the next targeted DRGs repeated the process.

CONCLUSION

Each resource management project requires sections of the processes outlined in these chapters. Methodically approaching various techniques for care delivery will result in high-quality performance at low cost to your department. The three areas to examine when considering throughput will help make the process seem less tedious. Becoming familiar with the subgroups and five performance parameters of case management will help you reduce the mismatch of patient needs and services while accommodating the increasing number of uninsured patients.

TABLE IV.6

Productivity Opportunity Roll Up

Community Hospital	Sept YTD 2010					Budget 2010				
		FTE Opportunity		Salary Opportunity			FTE Opportunity		Salary Opportunity	
CC Description	FTEs	Top Quartile (25%)	Median	Top Quartile (25%)	Median	FTEs	Top Quartile (25%)	Median	Top Quartile (25%)	Median
INPATIENT NURSING UNITS	208	27.0	18	2,637,912	1,709,519	230	44.7	34	4,604,611	3,542,274
EMERGENCY SERVICES	47	0.3	-	27,478	-	47	2.0	-	203,053	-
SURGICAL SERVICES	41	10.0	6	942,124	590,851	42	12.1	7	1,321,774	901,443
CARDIOLOGY SERVICES	12	3.3	2	335,483	254,487	14	4.7	4	524,964	428,811
IMAGING SERVICES	28	10.2	8	901,423	660,786	28	11.8	9	1,134,433	895,794
RADIATION THERAPY	10	-	-	-	-	10	-	-	-	-
LABORATORY RELATED SERVICES	29	7.7	5	-	-	35	11.6	9	-	-
RESPIRATORY SERVICES	12	-	-	-	-	14	-	-	-	-
REHAB SERVICES	39	7.9	4	643,829	344,260	36	8.9	4	699,714	333,519
Outpatient Clinics	23	7.2	4	482,600	275,238	43	15.7	13	944,764	780,426
MISCELLANEOUS ANCILLARY SERVICES	64	8.1	1	696,569	122,985	79	15.4	6	1,450,182	591,273
SUPPORT SERVICES	123	33.2	20	1,706,628	914,861	128	35.6	21	2,018,587	1,097,098
FINANCIAL SERVICES	23	6.0	2	268,458	110,491	26	8.1	4	381,442	202,680
ADMINISTRATIVE SERVICES	27	12.8	10	1,343,513	1,131,456	27	13.1	11	1,572,462	1,344,000
Non-Benchmarked Cost Centers	26	-	-	-	-	33	-	-	-	-
Zero FTE Cost Centers										
GRAND TOTAL	711	134	80	9,986,017	6,114,933	793	184	122	14,855,985	10,117,318

Note: CC, complications and comorbidities; FTE, full-time equivalent; YTD, year to date.

TABLE IV.7
Nonlabor Savings Matrix

Area	Initiative Name	Identified Spend	Low Recurring Savings	% of Spend LOW Savings	High Recurring Savings	% of Spend HIGH Savings
Surgical Services	Mesh	$394,875	$42,318	10.72%	$85,032	21.53%
Surgical Services	Heart Valves and Annuloplasty Rings	$534,530	$38,608	7.22%	$97,126	18.17%
Surgical Services	Orthopedic Total Joints	$5,322,161	$278,054	5.22%	$785,937	14.77%
Surgical Services	Shoulders	$224,020	$1,517	0.68%	$6,214	2.77%
Surgical Services	Spinal Implants	$2,641,248	$240,125	9.09%	$906,234	34.31%
Surgical Services	Suture Utilization	$478,371			$10,798	2.26%
Surgical Services	Suture	$478,371	$47,796	9.99%	$61,359	12.83%
Surgical Services	Instrument (Replacement)	$699,260	$144,778	20.70%	$284,630	40.70%
Surgical Services	Instrument (SMS - Repair)	$265,585	$69,926	26.33%	$100,293	37.76%
Surgical Services	Mammary Implants	$110,655	$3,677	3.32%	$10,350	9.35%
Surgical Services	Arthroscopy Supplies	$324,541	$0	0.00%	$31,119	9.59%
Surgical Services	Burrs, Bits, Blades	$605,957	$2,633	0.43%	$82,513	13.62%
Surgical Services	Ophthalmology (IOL)	$103,946	$8,892	8.55%	$17,719	17.05%
Surgical Services	**Reprocessing**				**$155,100**	
Nursing	SCD Sleeves	$214,518	$0	0.00%	$35,194	16.41%
Cath Lab - Radiology	Cardiac Rhythm Management	$4,870,807	$79,604	1.63%	$882,111	18.11%
Cath Lab - Radiology	Cardiovascular Stents - Drug Eluting	$1,427,350	$41,740	2.92%	$283,192	19.84%
Cath Lab - Radiology	Cardiovascular Stents - Bare Metal	$255,875	$71,423	27.91%	$114,320	44.68%
Cath Lab - Radiology	Contrast Media	$691,015	$20,730	3.00%	$55,281	8.00%
Cath Lab - Radiology	Isotopes	$885,529	$35,421	4.00%	$79,698	9.00%
Non-Clinical	Office Supplies (Formulary, Copy and Fax Toners)	$920,376	$55,223	6.00%	$101,241	11.00%
Non-Clinical	Housekeeping (supplies)	$627,798	$6,278	1.00%	$31,390	5.00%
Non-Clinical	Dietary - Catering	$100,188	$11,021	11.00%	$24,045	24.00%
Non-Clinical	Patient Food	$1,795,278	$125,669	7.00%	$233,386	13.00%
Non-Clinical	Dietary - Nourishment Products	$1,552,942	$108,706	7.00%	$201,882	13.00%
Non-Clinical	Employee Uniforms	$68,938	$689	1.00%	$2,758	4.00%
Non-Clinical	Meetings, Meals and Lodging	$421,722	$42,172	10.00%	$105,430	25.00%
Non-Clinical	Phone, cell/pagers	$8,487,964	$339,519	4.00%	$679,037	8.00%
Non-Clinical	Purchased Services	$1,763,206	$88,160	5.00%	$176,321	10.00%
Non-Clinical	Books, Dues and Subscriptions	$405,619	$40,562	10.00%	$101,405	25.00%
Non-Clinical	Equipment Rental	$486,297	$58,356	12.00%	$97,259	20.00%
Non-Clinical	Engineering Repairs and Maintenance	$1,892,193	$37,844	2.00%	$113,532	6.00%
Non-Clinical	Clinical Engineering Repairs and Maintenance	$871,272	$37,844	4.34%	$113,532	13.03%
Non-Clinical	Service Contracts - Clinical	$2,706,104	$54,122	2.00%	$162,366	6.00%
Non-Clinical	Service Contracts - Other	$161,219	$3,224	2.00%	$9,673	6.00%
IDENTIFIED SIU ASSESSMENT SAVINGS OPPORTUNITIES (To Date):		**$ 42,789,731**	**$2,136,631**	**6.85%**	**$ 6,237,477**	**15.88%**

Note: Cath Lab, catheter laboratory; IOL, intraoccular lens; SCD, sequential compression device.

173

The five steps in the Six Sigma process outlined in Chapter 9 will allow your department to continually improve. The resulting enhancements in performance will begin to effect other departments throughout your organization. Continued tracking will ensure that advancements in technology and patient acuity continue.

Development of team dynamics with clear and consistent communication is the most critical success factor. Using process maps to visualize patient flows and division of care by EOCs allow all team members to stay focused together on the reality of what is happening at the beginning of the project and can be used to track progress toward the end goals. Upfront analysis on DRG and both labor and nonlabor costs creates a baseline which can cover an entire system before narrowing in on first-targeted DRGs. Incorporating evidence-based medicine (EBM) to create pathways and order sets and then tracking using Six Sigma supports sustained results. Once the teams have been established and have gained confidence and success in the first round of efforts, speed and outcomes improve. Physicians are the only team members that may change from service line to service line as DRGs change. It is good to stagger rotation of other team members over the entire course of work. This is because the entire process covers the top 20% to 50% of all DRGs and can take several years. Once the structure and process is in place, organizations continue with the improvements as an ongoing process with reduced waste and costs while improving care delivery and patient and staff satisfaction.

Developing Leadership Skills

Nancy Bateman and Jacklyn Mead

People can be great leaders through vision and compassion yet fail because of gaps in communication styles, an inability to effectively manage time or confront issues and negative personalities. Many of the basic skills required for effective leadership, including the various management styles, are the focus of Part V. The discussion on team motivation and dynamics provides assistance for anyone who delegates responsibilities that produce results. In the discussion on communication and on time and change management, we review the details that successful leaders need to keep their department running efficiently. Working with others through conflict, general relations, and facilitated sessions also requires different methods of approach and conduct. Discussion on physician and pharmacy relationships and facilitated sessions conclude Part V. A final leadership skills case study exhibits the skills necessary for effective leadership in health care.

10

Developing Personal Management Skills

Nancy Bateman and Jacklyn Mead

This chapter supports the journey into management and offers recommendations and observations on what it takes to be a good leader. Before someone can be a leader, it is essential that he or she understands how to manage. Management of people is difficult because each individual is a complex combination of many personality traits, differing backgrounds, and general perspectives on life. Staff and personnel issues are commonly referred to as "HR issues"—meaning human resource issues that can take up a great deal of a manager's time. Helping staff members to perform at their best on a daily basis and working together as a team is the real backbone of leadership. The founders and background of numerous management styles are discussed, allowing you to decide which style works best for you. A successful leader motivates and inspires his or her team to perform without hostility.

LEARNING OBJECTIVES

1. Understand different management styles and recognize your own style.
2. List the qualities of effective management.
3. Understand what constitutes team dynamics.
4. Learn tactics for improved team motivation.
5. Understand the importance of communication timing.
6. Create an effective communication model.
7. Create your own time management log.
8. Recognize tasks that should be delegated to others.

MANAGEMENT STYLES

The first step in learning to lead effectively is understanding management style. There are many different styles of management, and these different styles all have the ability to reach the same levels of success. When a manager is confident and comfortable in his or her style, the manager can be as effective as possible. There have been studies throughout the years, and there are well-known industrial consultants who have developed their own theories on what are the best management styles. A few of the better known and successful business managers and economists from the early part of the twentieth century started to review how people worked and what motivated them to be more productive.

Scientific Management

One of the first methods adopted by the corporate world was *scientific management.* Developed by Frederick Winslow Taylor in 1900, this management style is sometimes referred to as "time and motion" with a stopwatch. Taylor believed that decisions should be made by management using a scientific method, which, in his theory, meant being unbiased. Taylor also believed the tasks for each job should be broken down into standard methods of completion so the workers could focus on the tasks and not have to make decisions on how to do the work. The model aimed to provide the right tools and incentives to workers for them to do their jobs. Taylor believed in matching the worker with the right skills for the required tasks. He also instituted pay incentives or bonuses for workers who increased their productivity (Taylorism, 2011).

Fayolism

Although Taylorism impacted the way floor manufacturing was managed, it was narrow in focus and by the 1920s a modified version of this management style was introduced by Henri Fayol. Also popularly referred to as *Fayolism*, this was a process of management versus a scientific approach to management. Fayolism became popular when he began to publish his ideas on organization and supervision of work. In his approach to supervision, staff needed to receive orders from one unit of command. In simple terms, managers were the authority and there was to be unity of direction, and individual interests were secondary to the common goals. Fayol instilled discipline into the work division and stability for the workers. Taylorism was dedicated to the efficient use of time and materials to complete each task and Fayol expanded on this to create principles for administration and the organization. Fayol also identified qualities a manager should have including characteristics of morality, general knowledge, health, and strong skills in the area managed (Henri Fayol, 2011).

The Hawthorne Effect

Another management style is the Hawthorne effect. In the 1930s, Elton Mayo conducted socioeconomic experiments at the Hawthorne Works factory to determine what factors would contribute to improved performance. The theory behind the experiments was that a happy worker was a better worker. In the experiments, he implemented several changes, including different schedules, differing degrees of supervision, financial incentives through overall production increases versus individual increases, and improved work environments. The workers were asked with each change how they felt the changes impacted their work. The results of the experiments found that workers felt valued by giving feedback on the changes and how these enhanced their work. Even more than pay incentives, improving work conditions had the greatest impact (Hawthorne Research, 2011).

Promoting a quality work environment and instituting shared governance contributes to job satisfaction and translates to better performance. The same outcomes of Mayo's experiments also appear to be behind the level of importance directed at patient, staff, and physician satisfaction scores on surveys.

Drucker's Management by Objectives

One of the more recent management styles was created by Peter Drucker in the 1950s. Drucker's management by objectives takes the results of the Hawthorne effect to a new level. The idea is to empower employees by clearly communicating to each employee what is expected of him or her and the objectives he or she is to achieve. The belief is that if every employee understands the objectives, he or she will contribute to the organization's achievements as well as to his or her own personal goals. This management style motivates individuals to set their own goals to meet the organization's objectives. An example of this would be to inspire each staff member to have a personal goal of delivering quality and attentive care to his or her patients in support of the organization's objective of high patient satisfaction scores. This also promotes the open door policy, improving communication and allowing feedback from staff, which supports an amicable work environment. The management by objective approach also created the SMART objectives for clarity of goals. SMART stands for

- S—specific
- M—measurable
- A—achievable
- R—relevant
- T—time bound (Peter F. Drucker, 2011)

This acronym can also be applied to project goals. Keep in mind that when focusing on goals, one should not forget to tie goals to outcomes. It is important to revert back to the basics of dealing with human beings when managing a staff. Consider the order of what is important to an individual. Maslow's hierarchy of needs is a helpful overview of the needs of an individual. Figure 10.1 is a high-level picture of Maslow's hierarchy.

Maslow believed that each person needed to have one level of needs fulfilled before he or she could focus on the next level. Physiologic needs are basic food, water, shelter, and clothing. Safety is next, then social needs, then esteem or acceptance, and finally self-actualization—meaning the individual is motivated to perform at his or her maximum potential. Maslow's theory is still considered relevant and studied in management today. Keeping in mind the five components and the order of their importance helps a manager to adapt staff needs into management decisions.

A good manager is flexible, anticipates the needs of staff, makes decisions, and takes advantage of opportunities when they arise. He or she is not afraid of confronting problems before they could threaten the effectiveness of staff.

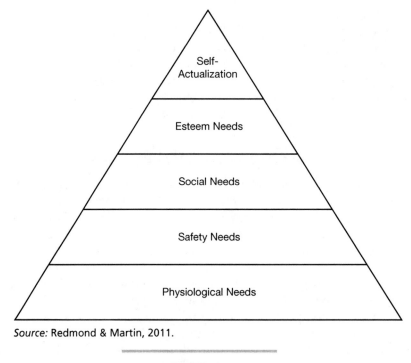

Source: Redmond & Martin, 2011.

FIGURE 10.1
Maslow's Hierarchy

The management styles described in this chapter only discuss a few of the theories that have been developed. However, there are a few management types that can create difficult situations.

TROUBLESOME MANAGEMENT STYLES

Long distance management is one example of a troublesome management style. If the chief nursing officer or department manager spends more time in the office and not among his or her staff, he or she is too far removed to know what is going on to support the staff and activities. Managers who are not familiar with the staff or must rely on other employees for basic operational understanding are often ineffective.

Insulation management is another type of management style that is equally ineffective and can even become destructive. The manager not only stays isolated in his or her office but also surrounds himself or herself with support staff that act as barriers between staff and the manager. These same managers have been known to use their protective staff as scapegoats when things go wrong.

The *repressed management* style is represented by individuals who may have been promoted without enough training or experience, lack confidence, or fear of being recognized as unable to do the job. Their lack of confidence prohibits them from seeing the project as a way to gain knowledge and skills. As long as people are willing to work together and are open to new ideas, however, everyone can benefit. These managers may be resistant to working with others, show their resistance and even slow progress, and stifle creativity.

Finally, the *hostile management* style is characterized by managers who suppress staff to the point of creating an unfavorable working environment. These managers either micromanage or can be disrespectful to their staff and peers.

Labels for ineffective managers may seem unkind, but recognizing the management style can be the first step in moving forward to establish a baseline and an understanding of the conditions in a given situation. Once personality and management styles are identified, the project framework can proceed with the most effective approach for success. The usefulness of knowing how people work and what makes them more productive can be analyzed and revised as more studies are done that reflect the current population. Being aware of established and progressive management theories are tools to enable you to create a management style that works best for you. A comfortable and confident manager is a successful manager.

TEAM MOTIVATION AND DYNAMICS

As previously discussed, mathematicians and engineers have used the word "sigma" as a symbol for a unit of measurement in product quality variation. Used in business, it is a way to identify any possible defects that prohibit a product from being absolutely perfect. By brainstorming anything and everything that could go wrong, teams are able to find solutions to problems before they even begin. By working backward through all of these problems, the product variation diminishes. In theory, a well-motivated and dynamic team can create a perfect business.

As a department manager it is important to use all available resources to create a motivated and dynamic team. The leaders of Six Sigma are an essential part of its methodology. Leaders must be responsible for implementing these processes. The use of the measurement and improvement tools is something that must be done by someone who is well trained. Communication skills are equally important. These skills allow the process to run smoothly not only with internal and external customers and suppliers but also with staff. This section is a guide for the methods of managing a successful team.

Before conducting a successful meeting, gather team members who are familiar with the processes and materials of a department. Target people who have shown that they are especially knowledgeable in certain areas and encourage them to be part of the team. Encourage anyone to attend, but individually talk to those who have something special to share, making sure they know how important their contributions are and that their assistance would greatly improve the quality of care patients will receive.

To get staff interested and willing to speak up about their favorite focus areas it helps to advertise. Find a place that everyone sees at least once during their shift: a bulletin board in the nurse's lounge is a great place to post announcements or agendas. Group e-mails, text messages, and social networking sites help advertise meetings as well. It is important to hold regular meetings at the same time and place. Assigning an odd time for meetings to start may also help people remember the meeting. Beginning on time is also critical. Subtly inform latecomers that their behavior is not acceptable by shutting doors once meetings begin. If tardiness continues to be a problem, present it to the group and see if they have any suggestions to help everyone arrive on time. Ultimately, speak privately to offenders and inform them that if they continue to be late, they will continue to disrupt the productivity of the group.

Try to keep meetings to a standard length so members can plan their schedules accordingly. People are more likely to participate and remain involved if they know there will be a set routine. As meetings become more habitual, attendees will also become more comfortable within the working environment. If there are many issues in a process that need to be resolved, try breaking them down into smaller and more manageable categories. Rather than hold a longer weekly meeting, try shorter daily meetings to progress through possible changes in procedure. Encourage meetings to move quickly while staying focused on accomplishing the most work in a short time. Stick to the agenda, but make sure it is flexible enough so others can ask questions or share ideas that drive to delivery. Providing snacks or other incentives at meetings is always an idea, but keep it simple. Request feedback or survey the group to see if anyone has any other ideas to make meetings more enjoyable and productive.

Strategies to Promote Motivation

To motivate staff members to get involved in a meeting, try some of the following approaches. When announcing the meeting, initiate a little preplanning by posting the topic under discussion. This can also be announced at the end of one meeting to provoke thoughts for the next one. By letting everyone know what will be discussed ahead of time increases the chance that resolutions will take less time to discuss.

The best way to get staff members to open up and share their ideas is to have the meeting leader do so first. Present an atmosphere of trust and model a focused, thoughtful working environment. Others will be more inclined to follow the lead and share accordingly. Ask people for their opinions; some people may be more reserved than others and need to be asked directly about what they think. Managers who are comfortable working with a team may overlook this nuance of human behavior. Never put down suggestions or ideas that someone has presented—being critical or not taking an idea seriously is a sure way to stop communication. Consider a suggestion or comment box to introduce topics for future discussions because this makes it possible to review suggestions later and allows those who are too intimidated to speak up to share their input. Try to keep the atmosphere calm, friendly, and relaxed, allowing everyone to be heard and take turns presenting information. Learn how to discuss issues in a fair way, where those with opposing opinions can compromise to create the most effective result.

Strategies to Keep Tasks on Track

Finally, make sure someone takes notes on progress. An idea that did not seem applicable at one time may be referenced again later for another topic. Having a record of meeting discussions can become an invaluable tool within a department. Post meeting minutes in the nurses' lounge so those who were unable to attend can be updated, and the meeting minutes may create new ideas for the next meeting as well.

To become a Black Belt leader of all department teams, it is essential to be familiar with the variances within Six Sigma. It is necessary to understand a problem in order to decide on a strategy or improvement initiative. Once there is a thorough understanding of defined objectives, one can organize one's team to create a solution. Being able to target individual strengths and weaknesses within a department creates a built-in resource for any number of problems.

Once everyone is assembled and aware of the meeting agenda, groups may be divided according to subtasks or assignments—this is where awareness of strengths and weaknesses is essential. Each group, or the team as a whole, should begin by brainstorming ideas and suggestions on possible solutions. Then, by working backward, teams can categorize, condense, combine, and refine their information. After regrouping, the information will then be assessed and analyzed in context with the main objective. Possible effects and results should be discussed at this point. Prioritize information and rank or list items according to their importance. Set a realistic schedule or plan of action that the team can implement. Finally, control and monitor the progress of implemented strategies. Progress will lead to perfection if Six Sigma methods are followed by a group that is motivated to perform and work together.

A *team* can be defined as two or more people who share responsibility for a common objective and whose efforts toward that objective benefit from coordination and communication. Teams should be consistently focused on finding the most successful method for delivering objectives. Additionally, teams should not be confused with workgroups, which do not work together toward a common goal because they are more segmented in their approach to improvement. Building an effective team is empowered by providing clear objectives, expectations, and parameters. Leaders should provide this necessary information as well as any necessary resources that assist in producing results.

Motivational Dynamics

There are many ways to get a team motivated to perform at their full capacity to solve a problem. One of the ways to organize motivational dynamics is by brainstorming. A *mind map* or *graphic organizer* is a diagram used to represent words, ideas, tasks, or other items linked to a central key word or idea. It is used to generate, visualize, structure, and classify ideas and as an aid in study, organization, problem solving, decision making, and writing. By beginning with a brainstorming session, issues can be better categorized and understood, making the most of available time.

Once the staff is motivated to become hardworking team members, it is time to discuss the dynamics within the team. Before meetings begin, everyone should know his or her role. A final outcome must be universally understood in order for the meeting to be successful. Begin by defining the reason for the meeting, making sure that everyone present is aware of the situation and ready to find a remedy. As a group, brainstorm or use some other form of organizational tool that initiates a plan of action, allowing teams to regroup easily according to their roles and responsibilities. Smaller groups can work together toward solutions that meet their individual team's goal. Analysis under different task forces can focus in many ways that meet the needs of the organization now and in the future. A problem can be organized in a discrete way where groups look at a particular failure in a certain process. This could be graphed using a pie chart to show various causes by percentage. Another group can create detailed flow diagrams to understand what is really going on in the process or subprocess. Delegating a set of people to map performance variations over time could become a continuous group always looking for new ways to improve.

Once breakout teams have analyzed information and discussed possible solutions, groups can reconvene and share findings. Presentations should be concise, yet detailed enough to promote total understanding among all participants. An affinity diagram is one method of capturing, analyzing, and organizing many different ideas, but there are many ways to deliver the information. Understanding how to create unity within the group so that the entire team complies with the vision is the most important part of management. Team meetings can be productive, informative, and fun as long as there is proper enthusiasm for a project and a willingness to work together.

Team members often have different viewpoints, and working together to try to achieve a common goal can be frustrating. To help the team realize that others may approach a situation differently, employ the following activities: Have everyone close their eyes and think of the days of the week. Have them assign a color to each day and write it down. Instruct them not to share their answers with anyone. Finally, share and compare the different color associations people chose for each day. Discuss why each person chose each color to better understand his or her process of thinking. Even if some people chose the same color, there will still be a different story to tell. Remind a team that if they can think of the days of the week in different colors, why not our work, responsibilities, and relationships? Seeing the days of the week represented as different in color makes it easier to imagine other more complex situations in different ways. Feel free to try other variations appropriate to a department. The aim of this exercise is to have colleagues recognize equally valid yet different points of view. The idea is to encourage the team to try to understand the views and ideas of others and incorporate them when making decisions.

Find a light, long object such as a stick, Hula-Hoop, or even a broomstick. The idea is that the object's gravitational force or weight is less than the collective force the team members will create. It must also be rigid enough so it cannot bend, yet not too heavy or it will outweigh the lift that the group size creates. Team members can be positioned in any way that works for them as long as their finger remains on the object. This can be done as a single group activity or smaller teams may be created. Teams of about five to six people are ideal. Instruct the team members to rest the stick on the outside, nail side, or back of their finger. Using one finger from each hand will increase the difficulty of the task. Positioning people on either side of the stick also increases difficulty. Having everyone press their finger down on a table or the floor for about 30 seconds before beginning can also trick the brain, providing additional challenges.

Ensure that everyone is in agreement on what is considered "the ground" before beginning. This is to make sure conflicts are avoided later. Once everyone has their finger in position, have them hold the stick about chest high. Working together, the first team to successfully lower the stick to the floor wins. If anyone's finger disconnects from the stick, the group must start over. It sounds simple enough, yet people will be surprised to see their stick rise to the ceiling. This is where teamwork comes in as everyone tries to figure out how to regulate the pressure, making the object descend rather than float up.

End-of-activity discussion questions may include the following:

- Why did the stick rise when we wanted it to go down?
- Did we anticipate the problem?
- How did we fix the problem?
- How did we feel when fingers lost contact?
- What are the effects of time pressures and competition?

- How might we coach or prepare others for this task?
- What have we learned about team working and problem solving?

Having the team go forward with their meeting with a heightened understanding that no two people think alike, and it takes teamwork to work through difficult situations, makes for a productive and happy group of individuals. Assigning any of these teams or small groups a defined failure as measured by Six Sigma analysts is sure to result in success. They should be able to work through any measured deviations to achieve total patient care and satisfaction. Using a varied number of combinations, utilize all team members to find the best strategies for all of the business processes.

Sharing results becomes the most important part of a meeting. It can be difficult to listen to everyone's conclusions at once and effectively incorporate it all into one process. Remember to look ahead for possible issues that may arise while implementing any new procedures or resources. Take the time to present solutions to these possibilities now, so if they do arise, a system or resolution is already in place. Whether the decisions revolve around sales, marketing, resources, or services, it is vitally important to the improvement of the business performance that suggestions and analysis be taken seriously.

Facilitating team changes can be as difficult as the decision-making process itself. New methods and products need to be implemented in the best way possible for patient care and cost-effectiveness. By the end of the meeting, teams should have a plan in place to implement newly created processes.

Change, or even the uncertainty of change, can be difficult for some people. Share potential roadblocks with the team that they may work through when implementing change. The following activity demonstrates how the brain reacts to change. Even having to accomplish a simple everyday task in a new way can be difficult. This activity is a great way to remind the team before sending them out on their own.

Choose any of the following basic tasks that work in an environment:

- Cutting paper shapes with scissors
- Tossing a ball of paper into a bin
- Typing on a keyboard
- Cracking an egg into a bowl
- Making a cup of tea, coffee, or a sandwich
- Writing or drawing
- Using a phone
- Putting a watch on the opposite arm
- Any task that involves counting, sorting, or building things (think playing cards)

Be aware that not all of these are applicable for the exercise, such as making a cup of tea blindfolded which may be dangerous. Observe and discuss how different people react in different ways to completing a chosen task under the following methods:

- Complete the task with a nondominant hand
- Blindfolded or with eyes shut

- Outside versus inside
- Perform the task in pairs when it is normally done by an individual
- Turn the task upside down to demonstrate strangeness, unfamiliarity, and relearning difficulties

No one reacts to change in the same way. Managers must have empathy for others, especially when managing change in their routine. Remind the group of how this exercise affected their ability to react to a certain task and how it differed from everyone else. This will help create a plan that introduces and trains employees quickly and easily.

Individual Motivation

Managers are often challenged with motivating a new or troubled staff member. The first step in supporting the staff member in improving his or her performance level is to observe behaviors and try to determine if this is a new and possibly short-term problem (such as a staff member with family problems coming to work late) or if it is a downward trend in productivity. With any problem, drilling down to the root cause is important. The cause may not be evident at first or even apparent to the staff member having the problem.

Establish root causes or privately discuss observed behaviors or improvements, and seek answers from the staff member. If the staff member is unwilling to offer the reasons for poor performance or did not realize that levels of output were less than required, the next step is to outline clear expectations and map out an improvement plan. Provide the staff member with a short time frame to show documented improvements. List three to five specific goals that will be monitored for a period of 3 to 6 months and meet with the staff member every two weeks to collectively review progress. If the performance improvement plan is not helpful, then further actions and involvement from human resources will be the next step.

Occasionally, the issue with a poor employee is a lack of confidence or training. Again, start with the root cause through a combination of observations and discussions. In the case of an individual who is struggling, assign him or her with a "buddy" who is an experienced staff member willing to support and guide the individual on a daily basis. In some hospitals, the education department offers special training for staff to function as a buddy or trainer for new hires.

Continuing Education

As a final component to team motivation, it is important to set an example to the staff by providing the best patient care possible. Health care is the industry of caring for patients, and a leader has the responsibility of keeping abreast of changes in health care delivery and regulations. It is imperative for the manager to set the example of continued education and ensure that the staff are also supported in expanding their knowledge. Health care changes rapidly and new technology comes into practice almost daily, so keeping up with all the changes requires constant effort and time.

White papers available on the Internet could be used for continuing education without the costs of seminars and are available for staff members on their own schedules. Organizations such as the Mayo Clinic and ECRI Institute offer current medical information and news on health topics. Subscriptions to organizations like ECRI offer recall notices and objective reviews of new technology and are great resources for white papers to distribute to the staff.

As a Nurse Manager, it should be a priority to stay updated on health news and encourage the staff as part of their annual reviews and certifications to stay ahead of changes in evidence-based medicine and clinical practice changes. The hospital compliance officer can assist with regulatory changes.

Some departments, knowing that staff time away from work can be too busy to add educational courses, offer monthly meetings so staff can share information and review literature on clinical changes. By using this method only one staff member needs to research new articles, and by sharing the reviews the entire staff, as well as patients, benefit.

Leaders are responsible for analyzing the labor and productivity of their department, continually finding ways to improve. Knowing where to make changes is not enough. A successful manager needs to know how to implement the process of change. Create teams whose members are knowledgeable of the processes and materials of your department. Motivate and lead them to accomplish goals that improve productivity. The information discussed in this chapter will help you develop your leadership skills.

COMMUNICATION

Communication is the most important skill for any manager. Staff, physicians, and supervisors all need to know the current state of plans for the department. Communication is not one-way; it can be ineffective or overused without a model that identifies who needs the communication, the form of communication for each audience member, and the timing of communication. Communication is best when it is consistent in its tone and delivery. The content of messages needs to be relevant to what each recipient needs to hear. In simple terms, the report delivered to a supervisor will be different from a report delivered to the staff. The level of what each group needs to hear should be reader specific and respectful of time constraints.

Communication takes many avenues: for ongoing updates to policies, any changes in process, or upcoming reminders, staff may prefer a weekly update posted in a break room and a mention of the content during weekly staff meetings. Reports prepared for administration need to be in greater detail with impacts, costs, and timing for each change implemented. Physicians need very short and easily accessible messages because they are often updated from numerous sources and their "need to know" may only include what affects them and where they can access greater detail if needed.

A new manager, leader, or health care provider must identify every party that requires communication. For each person or group, determine the best method of communication to reach them and use that way for them to reply or discuss messages. The timing of messages should also be set as soon as possible. Finally, the level of detail for each person or group should be determined.

When deciding on a plan for responses, comments, or requests for discussions, make it a simple task. E-mail is always a good source for reverse communication, but not all e-mails may be identified as connected to a communication report or memo.

If e-mail or a voice messaging service will be used to facilitate communication, make it clear that identifying subject lines or initial comments are needed. For those in a position of higher authority, where communications are coming through daily, consider a separate e-mail address for responses and replies connected to communications. Many large projects can be successfully controlled with a newsletter or website link so everyone interested in the project can access up-to-date information as needed.

Table 10.1 is a communication model formatted as an agenda used for a large nonlabor supply chain project.

Note that all people involved in changes are listed as to when they should receive information, how they will receive it, and in what forms. Messaging must be in several forms and should be repeated in order for the information to be accepted and retained. Planned schedules, whether for a large project or ongoing departmental updates, should be adhered to so consistency is maintained.

Notifying people who will be affected by changes early, such as staff and physicians, is important for two reasons. First, allowing them access to communication of planned changes, and then implemented changes, provides time for feedback and adjustment during the process. Second, the model begins to support the development of a habit among recipients so they know where to go to get information, and when they see changes, they are not caught off guard. Timing is also extremely important in communications. Knowing that the newsletter comes out each Monday or a staff meeting will occur each Thursday assures everyone that he or she will not be left out of knowing what goes on.

The same steps can be taken with all types of situations—from routine updates delivered within a single department to major institution-wide changes. The first step is to announce that communications about an update or change will be on the way, including who will receive messages, how often, and where the information will be available. For large projects, such as a nonlabor savings project, the launch should include notification to all involved parties outlining what the project is—or what communications are going to be offered—and how to communicate back to the leaders. A memo is often a good way to launch the model. A sample memo announcing a large project is shown in Figure 10.2.

Notice that the memo comes from the top of the organization and offers the avenue for feedback, describing and providing the duration (18 months) for the project. The memo should be e-mailed to all staff, physicians should receive copies in mailboxes, and it should also be posted on an internal website.

Along with a communication memo to notify involved parties of a project, a communication charter, as in Figure 10.3, is useful in providing clarity to the roles of the communication team and team members. Although it may be excessive for beginning routine communications within a department, certain aspects of the charter will be useful for more general planning.

Once all people involved have been alerted to the project, a schedule should be developed so consistent messages at the right level of detail and most effective mode are planned. All of the work completed in delivering information to the right people, at the right time, and with the right amount of detail, is only effective if communication starts early and allows those involved to participate in the information, even if it is only reserved to feedback or reaction to the updates.

Strong leaders bring in their staff and openly discuss planned changes before making decisions that could affect their staff. It is important to discuss plans with trusted

TABLE 10.1

Draft Products Communication Agenda

Date	Objective	Audience	Vehicle	Highlights	Person Responsible	Attachment
11/08/02	Launch communication team for supply chain products initiative	Corporate, administration, facility MM, department heads at all facilities	Letter or memo	Announce communication to team leader and members; list team's responsibilities, contact information, and method for submitting questions and/or comments	Letter will be drafted by XX and internal communications team and distributed through the CEO's office	A. Sample letter format
12/2/02	Formal launch to all employees of supply chain initiative	All employees	Newsletter, e-mailing, and displays	Publicize beginning of supply initiative; need for support and ideas from all staff; encourage collaborative efforts; provide answers to anticipated questions; identify basic agendas	Communication team with assistance as needed from supply chain team	B. Sample newsletter C. Sample e-mail memo D. Sample poster display
12/3/02 weekly	Update leadership group	Workgroup preparation	Issues tracking log	Weekly update of scheduled meetings, issues, and milestones	XX product specialist and communication team member	E. Sample issues log
12/8/02	Reminder to all employees: The initiative is still important	All employees with access to e-mail	E-mail memo	One or two short comments regarding efforts in progress	IS with script from communication team	C. Sample e-mail memo
12/16/02 bimonthly	Begin to actively involve all employees	Open to all employees, physicians	Forums	Representatives from facility teams available during lunch times to discuss progress/concerns; visibility	Supply chain, facility teams	None

(continued)

TABLE 10.1 (*continued*)
Draft Products Communication Agenda

Date	Objective	Audience	Vehicle	Highlights	Person Responsible	Attachment
12/16/02 monthly	Update staff and physicians on work in progress; successes; provide information supportive of changes	All employees, physicians, administrators	Newsletter	Product changes; provide product information as needed; recognize department "champions"; recognize individual employee suggestions implemented; provide feedback to questions and concerns received; may also include timely article excerpts	Communication team with information obtained from supply chain team and others	B. Sample newsletter
As needed	Updates specific to groups effected	Dependent on information or efforts needed	Memos; department medical staff or management meetings	Invitations to specific meetings with agenda (medical staff meetings); presentations to department, medical staff, or management meetings regarding specific needs	Information assembled and formatted by communication team and delivered by members of supply chain team	F. Sample invitation to medical staff meeting regarding orthopedic implant vendor selection
Monthly	Updates specific to groups affected	Dependent on information or efforts needed	Bulletin boards	Highlight product comparisons showing similar features; any differences and savings associated with change	Supply chain and facility teams	G. Sample board content
As needed	Buy in for new product groupings	Dependent on information or efforts needed	Product fairs	Hands-on display of new products with vendor samples and training	Communication team with vendor participation	

Note: MM, materials management; IS, information systems.

To: List Department Heads and MM Directors

From: XXX, CEO
          XXX, CMO

Subject: Supply Chain Initiative

I would like to introduce the members of the communication team who will be responsible for the distribution of information relating to the supply chain initiative. There is an urgent need to reduce product and service costs throughout the XX Medical Center (XXMC). Our ability to successfully address our financial imperative is largely dependent on all affected parties to become aware and to participate in a number of various initiatives that have begun and will continue to roll out over the next 18 months. It is essential that all staff actively support and contribute to each initiative when called upon to do so.

The members of the communication team are as follows:

XX, Department of Education
XX, VP of Surgical Services

Responsibilities of the team include the following:

- Provide timely, relevant information regarding progress of the initiative
- Maintain communication avenue for questions/concerns/feedback
- Notify appropriate personnel and medical staff of upcoming meetings

Reports will be delivered in the form of memos, weekly e-mailings, a monthly newsletter, and additional activities planned to include employee forums and product fairs.

Questions may be submitted to the Product Hotline (XXX-XXX-XXXX), in writing or through e-mail to the attention of XXX (designated contact person)

This is a project, which concerns us all and will significantly impact long-term viability of the organization. Thank you in advance for your cooperation and assistance as requested for this important component of our goal.

Sincerely,

XXX, CEO, XX Medical Center

FIGURE 10.2
Sample Memo

colleagues and weigh the changes with the impact resulting from the changes. Often, there are positives and negatives with changes, and as long as it is understood what the changes will involve, decisions will stand and be implementable. Consulting colleagues and staff is especially important when changes in the use of products are made or changes in policy or process are made, because safety issues may come into play.

- Clarify the importance of implementing supply cost savings—its objectives, aims, and expected outcomes in ways that will optimize understanding and enhance commitment.
  - Provide consistent messages to all audiences, including unique messages of emphasis to targeted audiences
  - Provide timely, relevant, and honest information
  - Help inspire motivation, enthusiasm, and participation in the process
  - Provide mechanisms for asking questions and getting honest answers from both within and outside the medical center
  - Provide progress in meeting time lines
- Provide the workgroup committee and project teams with a flexible response mechanism to handle challenges or issues.
  - Help coordinate with other initiatives as appropriate
  - Define the mechanism and supporting tools for addressing resistance
  - Identify communication roles and responsibilities
- Provide stakeholders with just-in-time information, which is specific to their needs.

ROLES AND RESPONSIBILITIES
Communications Team

- Plan organization-wide communications related to supply cost reduction implementations, including a communications framework of audience/constituency group, message, communication vehicle, and timeframe/frequency
- Provide feedback between the organization and project management and/ or workgroup; work with project teams and project management to develop, review, and participate in delivering formal and informal communications regarding implementations
- Identify obstacles and develop recommendations to build and develop an internal climate that encourages teamwork and is receptive to implementation efforts
- Serve as leaders in championing change throughout the organization
- Direct marketing, communications, and other production staff as to what materials to produce ensuring that production is completed on time, monitoring compliance with the communications plan

Project Management

- Provide input and approve the communications framework
- Provide resources to support the communications process
- Monitor the communications process through the communications team
- Assure compliance to the communication process

Project Team Members

- Provide input to communications team regarding communications framework: audience/constituency group, message, communication vehicle, time frame/frequency, and messenger
- Provide progress updates to communications team

FIGURE 10.3
Sample Communication Charter

Coordinator (Member of Communications Team)

- Schedule communication activities
- Assure adequate lead times in planning and preparing communications
- Mobilize resources
- Monitor execution of the communication activity
- Determine if the communication activity is effective
- Facilitate changing the communication plan with the communication team through the project management team

Graphics

- Provide a professional, consistent look for all communications
- Coordinate production of publications
- Assure adequate turnaround times for articles

COMMUNICATIONS

Audiences

- All employees and volunteers
- Management
  - Clinical
  - Nonclinical
- Senior management
- Project team members
- Users

Vehicles

- Employee forums
- Posters
- Newsletter (biweekly)
- Internet postings (monthly)
- Department staff meetings
- Management meetings
- Memos
- Nursing summations (quarterly)
- E-mail
- Paycheck stuffer
- Bulletin boards
- Brochures (include paycheck)

FIGURE 10.3 *(continued)*
Sample Communication Charter

People can be overloaded with trivial information, which can create the possibility that an important announcement can be overlooked. Keep in mind what mode of communication is required for different types of updates and reports. A department manager who is constantly e-mailing his or her superior with daily updates will be less effective when an important issue comes up. Respect other people's time and deliver clear, consistent, and succinct information when required. Communication is not one way. Be clear and consistent in your tone and delivery, and make sure you are listening and open to feedback. Reference the communication models in this chapter when evaluating your communication leadership skills.

TIME MANAGEMENT

One of the biggest challenges for most people is time management. Everyone needs to understand how to manage the time he or she has, prioritizing short-term and long-term tasks and goals in order to succeed. In health care, daily workflow can be interrupted at any time. As a manager, organizational skills and delegation of duties are not enough to stay on track with individual responsibilities. Develop a personal strategy and be willing to adjust the plan as needed. The ultimate goal is to fulfill responsibilities on a daily basis in a productive and effective manner to achieve success. Develop a plan and master necessary skills so that goals can be accomplished and a good model can be set for others.

When evaluating personal time management skills, it is helpful to start with a list of responsibilities. Include personal as well as professional responsibilities so all of life's tasks can be accommodated. Once everything is listed, keep a log of these responsibilities and what may cause problems or disruptions. Listing what has interrupted a routine, or what has caused delays, makes it possible to see what could have been prevented or what corrective action should be taken in the future.

Examine the list of responsibilities often and prioritize them. For repeating tasks, determine what is most important to finish during the day, week, or month. For health care providers, the list may include how many patients must be cared for, what staff reports to a manager, whom managers report to, and what daily tasks must be completed each day. Examine what time frames are involved and their deadlines. This helps to track work and prioritize each task.

Keep a log of what must be done daily, weekly, monthly, and long term. Add in unusual tasks that enter into the mix, then log issues and disruptions that arise when accomplishing the tasks for review later. This strategy may help when reporting outcomes to superiors, as well as help develop better skills for the future. Add ideas to try to improve personal workflows—these may turn out to be good ideas that can be shared with others. Be sure to list any problems encountered, which could reveal a pattern, making it possible to focus on the repeating problems to find the underlying cause. When reviewing workflow activities, it is also helpful to add external components, which interact with personal tasks under each item.

Develop a personal approach to managing tasks and time and know that lists and plans must be flexible to be effective. Reprioritize the list, reviewing the components and separating them in order of importance. If the list must be changed, log the pros and cons of moving them in the order of importance. Sometimes, this may simply mean moving a task to the following day to assist another person with meeting his or her deadline. In health care delivery, the important considerations should be if a change produces a positive or negative impact to patient care or will the reorder affect delegation of duties and reporting.

One of the most important guidelines to time management is to identify time wasters. Look over the list and evaluate each task to assess how much time should be spent on each item. List the activities that disrupt the prioritized list and which of these disruptions can be eliminated or performed differently or at a different time. Lastly, assess the list to determine if any of the tasks can be delegated to another staff member.

Once a plan for reviewing, prioritizing, and revising as necessary is in place, it is important to plan for interruptions. As an example, when a staff member comes in with an issue, ask, "Who owns this problem? Is it a managerial issue, a human resources question, or should the employee handle it independently? Is there another person who could handle the issue?" Evaluate the importance of the issue and if it should be handled immediately. When confronted with an interruption, consider if stopping to address the problem will contribute to accomplishing the day's goals. As a leader, the first priority is to the patients and then to the staff. The goal each day is to be a good leader and effectively manage the department. Determine if each interruption supports that goal or disrupts the ability to successfully fulfill the roles of a manager.

Time management is an easy goal to achieve by keeping to a routine of listing responsibilities, prioritizing them, and then managing interruptions. It gets easier to manage short- and long-term goals as good habits are developed. Skillfully leading your department in an effective manner that fulfills daily responsibilities should be your focus. Be willing to adjust your personal time management strategy to meet that goal.

11

Skill Development for Managing Change, Conflicts, and Relationships

Nancy Bateman, Daniel Edwards, and Keith Hanchey

When you're finished changing, you're finished.
—Benjamin Franklin

The successful Nurse Manager can manage change, resolve intradepartmental conflicts, and facilitate working relationships with many other department managers, including physicians and pharmacist colleagues. Change, of course, is a universal constant, but managing change is equally so and is vital to the success of the department and institution. The health care industry is continuously evolving. Hospitals place a high value on improvement, realizing that change is essential to forward progression. Conflict, another universal constant, requires the Nurse Manager to develop a management style that can minimize resistance and support satisfactory resolution to a group or individual conflict. Learning how to become a skilled session facilitator, whether as a speaker or as a meeting facilitator, is another invaluable tool. The session leaders' skills can help guide participants to a conclusion that can positively affect all of the participants and often also affect others outside of the core group.

LEARNING OBJECTIVES

1. Become familiar with different theories of change management.
2. Be able to recognize resistance to change and learn how to combat resistance.
3. Recognize how to work with the different types of conflict management.
4. Understand what nurses should expect from physicians and pharmacists.
5. Define and identify drug diversion.
6. Understand the preparation required for facilitating meetings of different sizes and purposes.
7. Learn effective ways to maintain the focus of participants during meetings.

CHANGE MANAGEMENT

People's reactions to change play a key role in understanding the change process. Every person will accept, adjust, and allow change to progress at his or her *individual rate of acceptance*. As part of the health care provider team, Nurse Managers face daily variances in staffing, product availability, and sudden life-changing events, both personally and those affecting staff members. Different situations and personality types respond to change from their own perspective, experience, and expectations. Whether the change is labeled as positive or negative, all change impacts everyone involved and demands energy and attention.

Managing the level of energy used to navigate through change is critical. Predicting when change will occur can be difficult—circumstances could relate to critical, unforeseeable, or opportunistic events. Understanding how people with differing personality types react to change can help prepare for implementing new processes. While in the process of managing a team going through a change, leaders will spearhead transitions.

Health care providers are familiar with managing tasks that focus on providing care for patients. When it comes to managing change, everyone uses a different set of techniques to manage issues, demanding one to think strategically, and anticipate issues and opportunities in a different process than with daily tasks. Managing change is not only about processes and steps, but it is also about how people respond, support, and maintain changes to achieve preferred outcomes.

Although models and theories are not absolute, understanding them and their foundations will provide the knowledge needed to deal with people's aspect of the changes being implemented. Change management is based on a system of understanding the dynamics and reactions to change people experience.

The Psychology Behind Change

Maslow's Hierarchy
Abraham Maslow's concept of the *hierarchy of needs* from his 1943 article, "A Theory of Human Motivation," helps illustrate the initial concerns and reactions people have to the news of potential change (Simons, Irwin, & Drinnien, 1987). This hierarchy was reviewed in the Management Styles section of Chapter 10.

Regardless of whether the change is positive or negative, others may feel threatened and fearful because of how they may be impacted. These first concerns and reactions are rooted in the "safety" and "belonging" stages of the hierarchy. Employees may have questions such as, "How will this change impact my current position and responsibilities?" "Will it impact my work relationships and people I depend on to help me?" Even the esteem stage can be impacted: "The new manager does not know everything I have done for our department" or "I was practically an assistant manager, now I don't know what role I will play, if any." Being aware of how employees may respond will help to bring them on board and support changes.

The Kübler-Ross Grief Cycle
The Kübler-Ross grief cycle, otherwise known as *the five stages of grief*, is a component of most nursing education. The Swiss psychiatrist, Dr. Elisabeth Kübler-Ross, was faced with the dilemma of managing dying patients who could not be cured. By studying

the grief process, she developed her model of the grief cycle of a patient's experience. Although the Kübler-Ross model is most commonly associated with the psychological responses to dying patients, healthy people experience similar reactions when dealing with lesser changes. In business and work situations, change may lead to a feeling of losing something or the perception of lost control. Being prepared for reactions to change by understanding their underlying stages, cognitive and behavioral reactions, are predictable from the start. Through communicating change processes from the beginning, managers can mitigate rejections and roadblocks. Consider the effects that changes will have and then stage the communication to have the desired impact, rather than waiting for a resulting disaster to what was a relatively simple change.

The Kübler-Ross Model of Grief

- Denial stage. Refusing to accept facts and information; avoiding the inevitable.

- Anger stage. Emotional stage often includes feeling frustrated. Once the realization that denial cannot continue is established, then anger sets in: "Why me?" "It's not fair!" "Who is to blame?"

- Bargaining stage. Searching for a way out. The hope that the individual can somehow postpone or delay the inevitable.

- Depression stage. Realization of the inevitable. The person begins to understand the certainty of what is going to happen.

- Testing stage. Seeking realistic solutions.

- Acceptance stage. Finally, finding the way forward (Shermer, 2008).

From a manager's perspective, the importance of the Kübler-Ross model is that it provides a scientific explanation of the expected emotional responses employees often experience after being informed of change, during the process of change, and in the final stages of change implementation.

Change Theories and Models

Lewin's Change Model

If you want to truly understand something, try to change it.
—Kurt Lewin

To be safe and belong are two basic human desires. All people strive for relative safety and the feeling of a sense of control. Through safety and belonging, people attach a sense of self-identity to their environment, which can be disrupted by the smallest change. Relationships, processes, and a sense of routine help foster security within environments. This sense of routine and stability is usually a roadblock, even when dealing with change that provides obvious benefits. Lewin's change model provides a system approach to disrupt a current state and move into a new, changed state.

Lewin's change model is the proposition that human behavior is the function for both the person and the environment. This means that one's behavior is

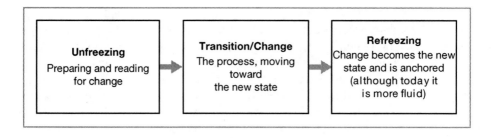

FIGURE 11.1
Lewin's Change Process

related to both personal characteristics and the social situation in which one finds oneself.

Within change management, Lewin's field theory is referred to as Lewin's change process or Lewin's model of change. Figure 11.1 summarizes the process.

Unfreezing
The goal of unfreezing (the first stage in Lewin's change model) is to motivate people to become ready and willing to begin the first step of change. The object is to unfreeze the status quo: the way everyone has always done it, made it, or said it.

Techniques
Starting the "unfreezing"

- Burning platform—critical crisis mode; do or die
- Challenge set goals—motivate them to achieve greatness
- Command—direct execution and instant
- Evidence—prove it with data
- Destabilizing—disrupt the safety zone
- Restructuring—redesign the organization to force behavior change
- Group dynamic planning—group brainstorming and planning sessions

Transition/Change
Once a team is on board to accept change, the transition stage can begin. Each stage is not necessarily independent, but part of a journey toward the new frozen state, the new status quo.

Techniques
Keeping it all going in "transition"

- Challenge set goals—motivate the team to achieve greatness
- Coach and educate—morale and knowledge building
- Facilitate and command—use a facilitator to lead the way

- Inclusion and champions—develop participation and internal leaders in the process
- Management by objectives (MBOs)—tell people what to do, but not how
- Open space—people talking about what concerns them
- Reeducation—train staff in new knowledge/skills
- Restructuring—redesign the organization to force behavior change
- Shift and sync—change a bit, then pause and restabilize
- Spill and fill—incremental movement to a new organization
- Stepwise change—breaking things down into smaller packages
- Whole-system planning—everyone planning together

Refreezing

The final stage is refreezing. The goal of this stage is to establish the foundation of the change into a stable and productive state.

Techniques

"Refreeze" the productive and stable state by:

- Burning bridges—ensure there is no way back
- Evidence stream—show them time and again that the change is real
- Golden handcuffs—put rewards in their middle-term future
- Institutionalization—building change into the formal systems and structures
- New challenge—get the team to look toward the future
- Rationalization trap—get them into action then help them explain their actions
- Reward alignment—align rewards with desired behaviors
- Rites of passage—use formal rituals to confirm change
- Socializing—build it into the social fabric (Straker, 2006)

Sticking and Cycling

An issue with the change process is the risk of sticking or cycling in one phase. This often happens when past attempts to change have failed. Staff can become stuck in a step and deny that true change will take place. The future to them may be going back to the old ways, it will only take time to go through this process the new manager or leader wants to "try." The lack of progression to the next step is not the only issue, but also going in cycles between process steps can be a destroyer of change. Stakeholders who are implementers can move forward too soon, while a past action is not completed, then have to go back to complete the previous step. This causes the process cycle to take longer and potentially derail.

Kotter's Eight-Step Change Model

John Kotter, a Harvard Business School professor, has written extensively on the topic of change management. He attained his experience and developed his model by studying the progress of hundreds of major companies, all which desired to "remake themselves." Kotter's basic model for change suggests that organizations should address the following steps:

1. Increase urgency for change
2. Build a team for change
3. Construct the vision
4. Communicate the vision
5. Empower people to act on the vision
6. Create short-term goals
7. Be persistent
8. Make the change permanent (Kotter, 1995)

The first step is to create urgency for change. Convince the employees that change is vital to the survival or the improvement of the company. Ideally, a manager should assure the staff that the change is possible without impacting job security but never mislead them. If there is a possibility of a layoff, explain that management is doing everything possible to make the financial changes necessary prior to consideration of a reduction in labor.

The second step is to build a team for the change. The team should also include at least one individual who will be a "hard sell." Once that person is on board, the team will have a powerful champion. If the change crosses multiple areas, create multidisciplinary teams.

The third step is to create a clear objective, detailing how the improved state will be better than the current situation.

The fourth step is to communicate this vision, which can kill or keep a change idea. Communication is the key in change management. For changes to succeed, staff must have a clear understanding of the goal because this gives them time to adapt. Problems arise when leaders have months to decide on a direction, and then try to implement change with lightning speed. However, this may have its place depending on the issue the change is needed to address.

The fifth step is to empower employees to execute changes. This can best be achieved by setting goals for interim steps, which lead up to the final state of change—the new status quo. The use of short-term goals (sixth step) assists the teams and employees to accept the change and gives everyone visual markers for progress. Using short- and long-term goal rewards can help make the change process fun, giving the staff a feeling of involvement.

The seventh step is about consolidating improvements up to this point and encouraging more change while acknowledging short-term achievements. The eighth and final step is to make the change permanent while integrating the new state within the company's culture (Kotter, 1995).

Summary

The personal aspect of change management can be described as the most important to understand and work through. It will include the emotions and opinions that will be faced when presenting new ideas to groups. Being prepared for how people typically react to change is essential to move past the first stages toward the transitional stage. Organizing clear directions are essential while ensuring that others know the vision for the final new state. By understanding how people react to change, a leader is not only responsible but also able to help others transcend to self-actualization. Whichever theory you choose to focus on, the psychology of change is a skill necessary for effective leadership.

CONFLICT RESOLUTION

Developing a proactive conflict management style is important because a leader will often encounter resistance to change or compliance. Using prepared techniques will support corrective action as soon as conflict occurs because leaving resolution to a later date only intensifies the issues. The first step in the process is to identify an individual style of conflict management. Once a personal style is established, it is possible to articulate a "win–win" strategy for resolving conflict situations. This prepared style will need a list of options and approaches to proactively manage conflict because each conflict will be handled with individual approaches.

To begin, it is important to review different types of conflict management.

- **Avoidance**. This style assumes that conflict is neither a danger nor an opportunity. These individuals may have little concern for themselves or others or the subject of conflict. Strategies for avoidance are denial, withdrawal, or postponement.

- **Accommodate**. In this style, the individual usually has low concern for his or her own feelings and has a high concern for the feelings of others. Often, this style is a "lose–win" situation. The individual may play down differences to maintain the relationship or the objectives of the conflict. People with accommodating personalities often assume the relationship might be sacrificed to get what they want.

- **Dominate**. This is definitely the "power" stance. Individuals with a dominate style will do what it takes to win and outcomes may often be a "win–lose" scenario. These individuals accept that the relationship must be sacrificed if they are to get what they want. Rather than give in, they will take over. Although the style seems harsh, this approach may be required in certain situations.

- **Compromise**. A more balanced approach where the individual is willing to trade off or "give and take." The person hopes each party can give up something to reach a resolution. In certain situations, there may not be a clear cut "win or lose" and this approach may be used effectively. The conflict is resolved if each party assumes they cannot both get what they want to the extent they want it.

- **Collaborate**. This style is confident and has high concerns for themselves and others. Individuals that tend to use this style like to explore the differences and interests of each party to the conflict. The individuals often will seek creative alternatives for the "win–win" scenario. They are goal oriented and strive to convey to the other party that everyone needs to work together to the common end result.

There are times when each of these styles need to be used and come into play for conflict resolution. It is not a matter of virtue, but rather a way of confronting conflict and using appropriate strategies to resolve issues.

One of the first things that must be done is to assign a level of importance to the conflict. Questions you can ask to help determine the level of importance include "Is this conflict life threatening?" "Is it a patient safety issue where a compromise might be dangerous?" or "Is it a conflict over delegation of duties or assigned overtime?" "Is the individual always late so the conflict arises when an annual review is performed?"

Start with the level of intensity and long- or short-term consequences and then assess the best strategy to use. Integrating styles and strategies to fit each issue is good for conflicts that are long term and when the parties will continue to work together in the future.

- **Avoiding.** This conflict style is most useful when the issue is something that will work itself out over time. In this case, the manager should discuss the lateness with the employee, with the understanding that the issue will be resolved. Sometimes the conflict is minor (interdepartment squabbles among coworkers) and does not require an intervention from management. This style should also be used with conflicts that are unable to be resolved. These may include personal values or societal issues.

- **Accommodating.** This style should be used to "smooth things over." Accommodating can be used to provide a temporary solution to an issue that can be dealt with at a later date or when there are other factors that will either resolve or move the problem to a higher level. Often, this style is employed when the issue at hand is of greater importance to the other party.

- **Competing.** When the goals of the issue raised demand immediate attention, dominating the discussion is required. Keep in mind that this may cause damage to the relationship, or in some cases, could end the long-standing relationship.

- **Compromising.** Finally, as in all conflicts when all parties are having difficulty moving forward, discussing a compromise may bring some resolution and satisfaction to all parties. This style is most helpful when the options to resolve the issues are widely divergent, or parts of the solution are unacceptable to each party. Discussing a middle ground may be the only acceptable choice.

A manager encounters resistance on a daily basis. Conflicts with change and compliance must be resolved quickly to avoid disruption of progress. By identifying your personal style of conflict management, you will be better prepared to resolve incidents professionally. Competent conflict resolution skills are essential for effective leadership.

PHYSICIAN AND PHARMACY RELATIONSHIPS

Effective communication is enhanced with an understanding of the roles and responsibilities of coworkers and colleagues. Two important groups that Nurse Managers interact with most are physicians and pharmacists. First, it is critical to know what to expect from physicians and pharmacists to enhance common efforts.

Physician Relationships and Communication

An important component to success as a Nurse Manager depends on the ability to communicate and build relationships with physicians. It is critical for Nurse Managers to make the effort to be out of their offices and in their departments while physicians are out making rounds and most accessible; otherwise, relationships will remain strained and ineffective.

Over the course of a career, Nurse Managers will rely on others to resolve many issues. A collaborative approach to care delivery allows for creativity and improved outcomes. The relationships will also increase staff and physician satisfaction because everyone's input is valued. Health care is a constantly changing environment, and physicians need to believe the department staff is there to work with them as integrated teams.

Physicians in the inpatient setting may be general practitioners, attending specialists, or hospitalists who take over for the care of a patient while in the hospital. Although hospitalists offer the greatest chance to establish strong relationships with staff, it is still important to reach out to all physicians in the community that may care for patients.

Today there are 954,000 physicians in the United States, of which there are 352,908 primary care physicians. This may seem like a large number, but this equates to an average of 1.25 physicians for every 1,000 patients. This figure varies from less than one to more than 1.5 physicians per 1,000 patients, depending on location (Sataline & Wang, 2010).

In the next 15 years, it is anticipated that there will be a shortage of 150,000 physicians (Sataline & Wang, 2010). In today's environment, current physicians are working harder because their reimbursements decline. A growing number of physicians are coming to hospital administrators asking to become full-time employees, even in community nonteaching organizations. In addition, patients admitted to hospitals today are sicker and require higher levels of care, which means that physicians are being asked to work harder while compensation continues to decline. Reimbursements did increase slightly in early 2011, but the increase was small compared to what was lost over the past 10 years ("Medicare Physician Payment Up Slightly [Again]," 2011, p. 14).

It is important to understand the situation physicians find themselves in because many changes are being discussed for the future of health care. Understanding the pressures and increasing workloads of physicians contributes to other staff members' need to reach out to them and offer as much assistance as possible. As all strive to deliver a better health care experience for patients, it is vital to work as a team as each role contributes to the quality of care provided.

With this situation in mind, there are several expectations that nurses and Nurse Managers should expect from physicians. To gain credibility and respect, nursing staff must demonstrate knowledge of the patient condition and be able to report on demand about the current status of the patient. In return, nursing staff should expect

- respectful dialogue between physicians and nurses regarding patient care
- answers to questions on care and order sets so there is a clear understanding of the intended outcomes of the treatment plans
- the opportunity to discuss care options as it relates to activities of daily living, discharge planning, and family counseling

- documentation that supports appropriate coding and clarity of patient condition
- the same level of knowledge of the patient condition and current status from the physician
- primary care physicians and specialists to communicate with one another so seamless and coordinated delivery of care is possible

It is critical to assess the level of collaboration between nursing staff and physicians to ensure that communication is effective and that the relationship is beneficial for everyone, including patients. If communication is one way with the physician dictating orders, interaction is limited. Remember the third party to the team approach is the patients themselves. Once the physician leaves, the patient needs to be able to ask questions related to his or her care. If the nurse is only performing the ordered tasks and has no idea of the future plans or cannot offer insight into the reasoning behind the orders, then both the patient and the caregiver are working with limited sight.

Hospitals should offer patient rounds where a diverse group of staff can review a patient's care and offer open communication from all disciplines on how best to treat the patient. This is the most ideal example of communication because all team participants are able to contribute their areas of expertise and, collectively, the patient has the benefit of all resources. In the past, management of a patient rested entirely on the opinion of the physician. As health care has evolved, all caregivers have become involved in the patient care decisions. The basis for all of these changes is improved and respectful communication.

Pharmacy Relationships and Communication

Today's Contemporary Health System Pharmacy Service

Hospital pharmacy as practiced in systems, community hospitals, and academic medical centers has evolved to become a clinical department with a very large supply chain component with the department's drug budget or drug spend making up between 75% to 85% of the total budget. Agents are becoming more complex in their chemical makeup and are more expensive.

The major focus of a pharmacy service is to manage a formulary to use in the organization for the treatment of its patients as approved by the medical staff governance, to control the distribution of the drugs for safe and efficacious use, to maintain the regulatory controls dictated by state and federal laws, and to oversee the safety of every patient receiving drugs within the organization.

The education of pharmacists has changed over the years to become more clinically focused as the degrees are called PharmDs. The training includes pharmacology, therapeutics, and clinical residencies that specialize many of these practitioners beyond an undergraduate degree. The educational programs are 6 to 7 years in duration with accredited residencies and fellowships beyond the PharmD.

Some of the clinical services that are well established within health systems include, but are not limited to, medication reconciliation upon admission, medication discharge counseling, antibiotic stewardship and dosing programs, total parenteral nutrition (TPN) prescribing, research, and patient and staff education.

Nursing Leadership Expectations

It is advised that there be a very close relationship between pharmacy and nursing beyond the distribution and easy access of drugs for nurses to administer to patients. The following categories are suggested as basic expectations.

Nursing Expectations

- Accuracy
- Pharmacy reconciles the medication administration records (MARs) with the chart
- Patient allergies are screened and communicated to the prescribing physician if drug allergies are found
- Physician orders to be clarified by pharmacy if there are any questions regarding the order
- Oversight by the pharmacy that protects the safety of the patient and should also expect to be educated on any new medication that is being ordered by a physician
- All physician order entry sets are reviewed by the pharmacy and approved by the pharmacy and therapeutics (P&T) committee of the medical staff

Medication Administration Records

Many pharmacy computer systems prepare nursing MARs as a result of the order entry by pharmacists. Many systems are now preparing the MARs as a result of physician order entry. Safety and correct drug administration is the focus of the MAR. Complete documentation of the drug administered and recording of any observations as a result of the drug administration are also functions of the MAR and charting.

Patient Safety

Patient safety initiatives vary from organization to organization. Medication errors cause injury to patients in large numbers and many can be very serious or even fatal. Labeling is usually done by the manufacturer and has found to be confusing. Safety is a joint responsibility of all departments and every discipline in the hospital setting.

Nursing Expectations

- Stock drugs are labeled in a manner to call attention to high-risk drugs
- Pharmacy to provide orientation for new nurses around medication handling and drug administration
- Pharmacy to review and approve all drug administration policies and procedures
- Periodic continuing education and refresher courses on drug administration and the proper documentation procedures
- Alerts about side effects to observe and document for physician awareness or a policy in place to automatically stop therapy if the effects are threatening to the patient

State and Federal Regulatory Compliance

Drug diversion is a fact of life that every health care leader will deal with in today's practice settings. Pharmacy is responsible for policing drug diversion and is responsible to the state boards of pharmacy around the country. The state health professional licensure boards deal with drug diversion and addiction in enormous numbers. The pharmacy director is normally designated as the pharmacist-in-charge for the organization, which allows for the issuance of a pharmacy license to the organization. Without a state pharmacy license, the organization cannot be issued or maintain a federal Drug Enforcement Administration (DEA) license so as to acquire and use controlled substances, normally used for pain management.

If drug diversion is not taken seriously and addressed in a collaborative way between nursing, pharmacy, administration, and the medical staff, the organization can become at risk for loss of that DEA licensure. Addiction destroys lives and if nurses or other health care professionals are diverting drugs, innocent patients are put at risk. All of the actions regarding regulatory controls lie with the responsibility of the pharmacist-in-charge.

Nursing Expectations

- Zero tolerance of drug diversion
- Oversight of control substance handling and documentation
- Any irregularities sighted by one or more individuals
- Cooperation and investigation of discrepancies
- To be held accountable for observing erratic or suspicious behavior by nursing professionals and be expected to collaborate with the pharmacist-in-charge and appropriate executives in the organization
- Prosecution and notification of the state board of nursing of any drug diversion

Nurse Education

Drug therapy is becoming increasingly complex. Drug administration devices are becoming more complex. Pharmacy is the subject matter expert in drug therapy that resides in the organization.

Nursing Expectations

- Education of all new staff to drug administration policies, controlled substance policies, and charting responsibilities for drug therapy
- Alignment of nursing continuing education to educate nurses about new agents admitted to the formulary
- One-on-one education sessions for nurses not families with an agent or how to administer it
- Collaboration on any process that is preventing efficient and timely medication pass times, including where the drug is stored and the process to access the drug for administration

Understanding the role the pharmacist plays in the daily responsibilities allows the manager to plan for the avenues of communication and the timing. Build strong relationships with the pharmacy department and demonstrate awareness of their roles and the unique services that are a vital part of patient care delivery. Mutual trust is essential so that when issues arise, the discussions required to solve problems are entered into and completed with respect.

The pharmacy department is a clinical department where drug knowledge expertise and responsibility for regulatory and patient safety resides. The cooperation and collaboration between nursing and pharmacy is essential if the patient is the central focus of the organization. Drug distribution processes impact nursing time, which impacts patient access to the professional nurse and timely administration of the prescribed therapy.

Clinical pharmacy services enhance the focus on the patient when the drug reconciliations are done by pharmacy, when an antibiotic stewardship program is administered by pharmacy and vancomycin and aminoglycosides are dosed by clinical pharmacists, and when discharge counseling of drug therapy is done by pharmacists. The nursing/pharmacy team creates a practice model that protects patients, protects health professionals, and provides good outcomes for the patients and the organization.

Being able to communicate with physicians and pharmacists is essential for productive nurse management. Knowing what to expect assists in enhancing common efforts. Use the communication model in Chapter 10 to ensure the process is clear and consistent between your department, pharmacy, and the physicians. Building relationships with others promotes a more effective working environment. Take the time to understand the position of others.

FACILITATED SESSIONS

One of the most recognized leadership skills is the ability to deliver a speech or manage discussion during a meeting. Facilitated sessions are a form of meeting where a leader helps guide the participants to a conclusion that affects all of the participants and often also affects others outside of the core group. Throughout the rest of this chapter the focus will be on general speaking and meeting leadership, and on larger group discussions where the main role of the leader is to keep everyone focused and working toward a collective outcome.

There are many resources and training programs to help a new leader become a good speaker. Two of the most important aspects of a good speaker are giving a genuine presentation and practicing often in front of crowds and committees, delivering components or entire speeches. While watching other speakers can be helpful, it is important to find which techniques personally feel most natural and make it possible to deliver the message confidently and clearly. Reviewing the speech on film is a helpful technique and can be a great method to pinpoint ways to improve. Above all, the most important part of delivering a speech or facilitating a large workgroup is to prepare and know the content.

The following is a discussion of different presentation types and the use of aids such as PowerPoint slides, lecture podiums, and facilitated sessions.

Simple Presentations: Delivering Updates and Necessary Information

Weekly department staff meetings and presentations to administration on monthly variances or performance updates fall into the area of simple presentations. The format of the meeting or presentation should be consistent. In this way, the messages are heard because the audience, whether one or 100, can focus on the message rather than adjusting to a new format.

Start each meeting by announcing what the update is about, even if the audience knows which topics are on the agenda. Never assume that the audience is aware of the meeting topic. The agenda for any update, however routine or casual, should start with the introduction: state the update, report, or presentation and then summarize at the end by repeating the points the audience should take away. This is especially important when the discussion is serious. Consider the example of a product change and how the presentation affects the use on a patient. The staff needs to be clear on the change because this could pose a safety issue. Any information that needs to be retained or accessed later also needs to be printed and distributed. If PowerPoint slides are used, the most important slides can be printed to deliver the information easily. If PowerPoint is not being used, make sure to keep handouts simple so the reader can glance at the handout and absorb the information needed. Audiences will appreciate the simplicity and clarity of the information they need to know.

Presentations, speeches, and lectures all require greater preparation, rehearsals, and some form of presentation medium. In today's world, the most common method is the use of PowerPoint slides. PowerPoint can be learned through a class or simply experimenting with the software accessing the help function as needed. Keep slides to a minimum and never use more content on any page that would require someone to take more than a minute or two to read. For presentations with the intent on delivering important changes such as product changes or policy changes, use one- or two-slide PowerPoint presentation, with bullets highlighting the most important information as handouts. Audiences need to understand the important components of the presentation, so keep it simple and clear.

In a more formal setting, where a process of detailed delivery is necessary, a full PowerPoint slide deck may be required. Start with the agenda for the presentation and keep the flow in a logical sequence. The slides should be in the background and have major points, whereas the rest of the information is presented in greater detail. If the slides are too busy to understand, or if the speaker is just reading from them, the audience will quickly resort to reading the slides and will not listen to the presenter. Another important point to remember is to move around a few times, possibly stepping up to the slide and pointing to a bullet to add emphasis to the fact. This keeps the audience interested.

Presentations using a podium can be useful if it is necessary to refer to notes because this allows the speaker to have the notes without holding them. While referencing notes should be kept to a minimum, it may be necessary to have notes available, especially when numerous facts are being delivered. When using a podium, pay close attention to the height because a podium can overwhelm speakers who are short in stature, making it difficult for them to be seen and heard. If the height of the podium is an issue, consider stepping just to the side so that notes will be available without overwhelming the speaker.

For all presentations, consider how movement will be used. It is essential to practice hand movements so that they are used in a way that naturally emphasizes the delivery. It is helpful to keep arms away from the body so that movements are slightly exaggerated. Keep in mind that larger audiences will require more exaggerated movements because the speaker is farther away in this case.

When acting as a facilitator for a large group, which can be anywhere from five or eight or up to 30 or more, the preparation work is intense. Given enough thought and preparation, the goals of the session will be met. A facilitated session is different than a design session, which many have experienced. A design session is much larger and occurs over more than a day or an afternoon. A facilitated session is a minor version of a full-scale design session. Facilitated sessions are very useful when developing an approach and work plan to implement changes using a large group of end users or stakeholders. A stakeholder is someone who will be affected by the changes and therefore needs to be able to have input into them. The plan to implement the changes happening must be discussed among the stakeholders, so the changes are more acceptable and sustainable.

The session may start out with a large group, and the reason, agenda, and goals for the session are presented to the entire group. Then, several smaller groups may break out and work on a segment of the agenda. At the end of the session, the breakout groups should reconvene and report the work they did to the rest of the participants. This is a great way to bring contributors together in 1 day or afternoon, so they can progress forward with ideas, solutions, and plans for implementing the changes that might have otherwise taken months of separate meetings to attain.

For a formal facilitated session, it is important to decide who the stakeholders are. Do not forget to think outside of the department and include physicians, considering if they would be impacted with any of the changes. Plan the date well in advance, so all invitees have enough time to add the date to their schedules. A letter or memo distributed to everyone at least two weeks before the event, with follow-up calls a week before, ensures everyone invited has every opportunity to attend. If the list includes physicians, make sure to offer them the option of contacting the leader, with their thoughts should they not be able to attend. Another helpful technique is to state in the invitation that changes will be decided at the meeting that may impact their work. This message alerts them to the importance of attending, or using the option of discussing their opinions with the leader beforehand to be incorporated into the meeting's discussion.

Keep the invitation short and direct to the point. State the reason for the event, the reason why the recipient is invited, and the goals of the session. When people begin to arrive for the session, the room needs to be ready. It is helpful to have posters and breakout sessions already set in the room, so that participants walk in and feel energized. Use a template and have it blown up and attached to the walls—one at each breakout area—so the participants have a consistent way to work through their assigned tasks and develop their plans of action. Before the meeting, assign the breakout participants. This technique maintains an orderly transition from introduction to working sessions. Each breakout team may assign their own leader, or this can be done ahead of time and help prepare the leaders with the flow and outcomes planned. A template similar to the one shown in Table 11.1 is helpful because it goes in logical order from what is currently happening to what the participants want or need to see going forward. It also covers what best practices are known about the goals in mind. Finally, it allows for a work plan with dates assigned to each task.

Notice that Table 11.1 includes a section to identify what risks may be related to the changes and the quantification of results. The quantification might be a dollar savings, an improvement in patient safety, or staff satisfaction. Every change should identify the risks, barriers, and quantifiable results that will be tracked for compliance or success.

TABLE 11.1
Work Plan Template

TEAM:

No.	Task Description	Weeks Ending	7-May	14-May	21-May	28-May
	Current state description					
	Leading practice opportunities					
	Future state description					
	Quantification and risk					
	Implementation plan					

Recall the MBO style popularized by Drucker and the use of SMART, which was outlined in the Management Styles section of Chapter 10. This method is a good list to use when designing and facilitating work groups. Outcomes of the session should be specific, measurable, achievable, relevant, and time bound (SMART).

Participants should have a clear understanding of what the expectations are for their involvement and have all material to be reviewed during the session available two days before. Begin the session with rules of engagement, which is a list that should be visible at the front of the room. The rules of engagement should include specifics such as keeping cell phones on vibrate, breaks will start on time and will end on time, be respectful of others, and allow them to voice their ideas without disruption. Also, have a flip chart at the front and label it "parking lot." This chart is used to capture ideas or issues unrelated to the intended goals and can be revisited later in a different session or forum. Documenting parking lot items keeps the momentum going on what is important for the day and still captures the remarks for later use.

At the beginning of the session, icebreakers are helpful. This technique was popular in the late 1980s and 1990s, but icebreakers still serve the important function of relaxing the participants and starting the session with a smile. The session needs to be productive yet gratifying.

The Fastest Finger Quiz, which mimics the game on television, is an example of an icebreaker. Try using a case study of a patient who is 70 years old and is in the hospital to undergo surgery, which can be useful during budget-related sessions. Four surgeries are listed. The audience has just a few minutes to list the four surgeries in order of least reimbursed to most reimbursed. The answers are then shown to the group and they get a second chance to do it again with the same patient but for different surgeries. Each time the answers are shown to the group, the reimbursement is shown alongside the actual costs of care for that patient undergoing different surgeries. The idea with this icebreaker is for the nursing staff to realize that the business of nursing requires quality and safe outcomes. The Fastest Finger Quiz in this case helps illustrate that all have an important part in delivering care with the least amount of waste while being mindful of the costs of care.

Another icebreaker that can be simple and fun is the use of colored candies. The teams are passed a bowl of colored candies and each participant is to select three. Once the candies are in front of all the participants, a chart is exposed to show what each color requires the person to do. Each participant may select one of the three colors and they have to answer the corresponding question. Often, participants will choose the same color for all candies, which means they do not have a choice in what they answer. Questions can be more personal and range from the most embarrassing moment in a participant's life to what would he or she do if he or she won the lottery.

Before breakout sessions are started, or in the case when the session is a smaller meeting and the participants can accomplish the goals on their own, a PowerPoint presentation allows everyone in the room to see and review the same material at the same time. As facilitator, it is important to include an agenda, goals of the session, and the current facts related to the intent of the session.

Additionally, an overview of the assessment findings should be shared with the group. Any significant data, such as products or process flows, should be enlarged and posted so participants can collectively walk through what is commonly called "current state." In many cases, a matrix with necessary tasks or elements of the situation at hand can be helpful because it helps all members of a team understand how their actions impact others. The matrix will make it possible for the entire group to discuss the situation to discover the best approach to the problem. The matrix shown in Figure 11.2 shows segmented tasks, listed with the positions currently involved in each step along the process. A list of what they were doing was also recorded.

After moving through the matrix, ask participants to move to their assigned breakout sessions so predetermined subgroup members can develop their own template. First, the groups are validated on what was recorded as their current state. The work plan templates should be filled with current state and leading practices, which allow the subgroup to compare their ideas to the organization's processes to leading practices.

The subgroups can then create what they would like to see as the new process and identify what skills should be used at each step. Keeping the roles and responsibilities to a list of skills, and not using names, allows participants to create

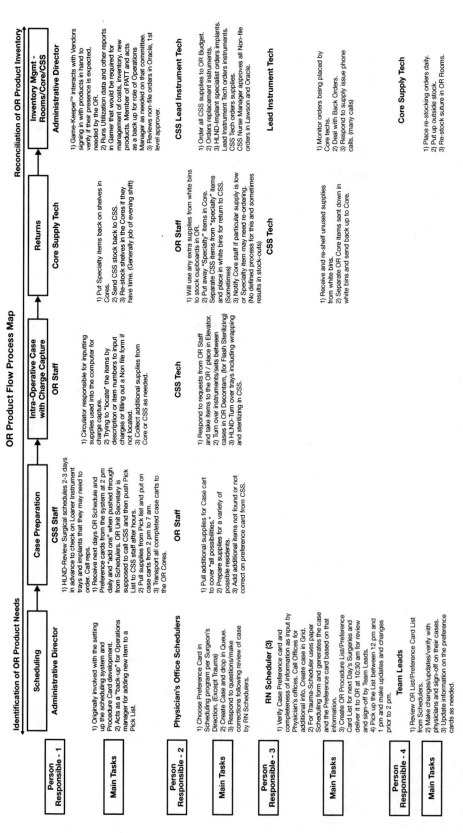

FIGURE 11.2
Task Matrix

Note: OR, operating room; CSS, central sterile services; RN, registered nurse; PATT, preadmission testing and teaching.

improved processes without interference of personalities or inferring that anyone who had previously been assigned to the tasks was not doing a good job.

The total process as shown in Figure 11.2 was broken down into:

1. Case scheduling

2. Case preparation

3. Intraoperative case product flow

4. Returns

5. Inventory management

Remember, staff members are busy and focused on what they need to do. It often takes an outsider to come in and look at the entire process to see where the breakdowns are occurring. In the consulting business this is referred to as using "fresh eyes." In all subgroups, representatives from all involved departments should be included. Real success often comes from different perspectives coming together with easy solutions—once each party understands how their contributions allowed the total process to be enhanced.

Once all subgroups have completed their work, the total group of participants should come back together, and a leader from each team can present their future state risks, quantified improvements, and work plans with timing to complete the changes.

Final Tips

The real challenge is to keep groups and individuals focused and moving ahead. Some people feel they are being attacked just because an issue that has occured in the area where they work is discussed. For these individuals, it is important to allow them a few minutes to voice their opinions or explanations regarding why the issue is occurring, but then stop them by respectfully interrupting their speech and make a quick summary of their statements. This does not embarrass them but allows the group to move on. If individuals begin to tire or start their own conversations, simply walk over to their area and stand behind them while continuing to facilitate the group. This usually draws attention to their disruptive behavior in a nonconfrontational way. In severe cases, it may be necessary to call them out and ask that the entire group listen and allow others to have the floor.

Continue to focus on the agenda and keep candy on the table or provide food at breaks so people can keep their energy levels up. Remember that your role is to keep everyone focused and working toward the collective goal. Being able to lead a group requires general speaking and leadership skills. Reference the tips and suggestions discussed in this chapter to ensure that your methods are productive and professional.

Conclusion

Nancy Bateman and Jacklyn Mead

CASE STUDY

As a summary of the skills necessary for strong leadership and management of staff, what follows is a case study of the management issues encountered in a community hospital that required extensive changes so it could financially recover and remain a service to the community. The organization was in a rural location and over an hour away from the next major hospital. The community was going through economic changes and many of the residents, having lost their jobs, were moving out to other parts of the state. This situation meant that patient volumes had declined and were not expected to return. To continue to operate as a full-service hospital, the executive management recognized that it had to reduce labor and nonlabor, and review all service offerings to determine what they needed to maintain in order to provide the best care for the community.

Once the data was collected and analytics completed, opportunities for labor reductions were available in almost every department. Some of the obvious choices for reductions in operating expenses were duplicated educational offerings that were also offered by the community college. Diabetic counseling, parenting classes, and art classes for occupational therapy were a few of the programs dissolved. Discretionary spending was also reviewed. Rather than to eliminate other jobs, these were areas that could be quickly eliminated until the financial situation stabilizes.

Within the reductions related to service lines, it was determined that elective pediatric cases would be sent to the larger city hospital because the volume of elective cases was so low the nurses could not maintain their certifications.

During the project, all efforts were made to reduce supply costs and review service lines that were not profitable. When it came to reducing staff, the skills of the management team were critical in achieving the goals. Almost the entire staff had worked there for their entire careers. All of the department managers had advanced in their careers while working at the hospital. The manager of the emergency department also had a sister working at the hospital and the chief operating officer's wife was a nurse there. Everyone was not just a colleague but a family member, neighbor, or Boy Scout leader to their sons. The vendor community for supplies was mostly local and had family and friends tied to the hospital.

To reach the labor reduction goals, the process had to involve meetings with each department manager to work through the reductions. The approach used was the flex staffing model, as described in Chapter 2, and core staffing had to be reduced to the bare minimum while expanding the float pool and sharing staff across the system so that fluctuations in patient volumes were handled safely. The variance in response to the project was significant. In some departments, the managers cried through the meetings. Others became very angry and screamed that the reductions would cause harm to their patients, despite a high ratio of nurses to patients.

When a project like this occurs, a great deal of education needs to be included for management training. Due to years of overstaffing, the staff did not have any specific staffing model in place or staffing grids related to census. No sitter polices were in place because there was always a supply of nurses available to provide the service.

The first step in the process was to establish what the average census per department had been over the past 12 months and map out the trending by department because it related to reduced patient loads. A simple tracking tool was developed so each department could flex up their staffing as needed, versus the usual flexing down of staff. In most cases, managers send staff home when the census is low. For this hospital, base staffing was established; the float pool was expanded to flex up as needed.

The project required an additional four months of work to reduce the levels of staffing and educate managers on how to effectively run a department. As most of the managers had no specific management training, a minimum of two months included classroom education on leadership, budgeting, and other critical skills.

CONCLUSION

Informed and adaptable management is a critical role in the overall viability of an organization. When economic times create challenges, all skills will be tested. Staying true to a personal management style and keeping focused on patient care delivery, as well as the needs of staff, will make it possible to navigate the roadmap toward success.

Choose a management style and stay with it. Consider the dynamics of the team and use various ways to motivate it to accomplish goals thoroughly and collectively. Communicate all changes and relative information to anyone who may be affected. Manage time effectively by making lists and considering what distractions or tasks may distract from goals and responsibilities. Diffuse any possible conflicts before they interfere with progress by following the advice in the Conflict Resolution section of Chapter 11. Foster good working relations with the pharmacy department and the physicians themselves. Finally, facilitate work sessions in an organized and productive manner. Modeling professionalism, knowledge, and an understanding of the newest methods in health care will inspire the team, while leading a department that operates efficiently while continuing to improve.

References

Aiken, L. H., Sloane, D. M., Cimiotti, J. P., Clarke, S. P., Flynn, L., Seago, J. A., . . . Smith, H. L. (2010). Implications of the California nurse staffing mandates for other states. *Health Services Research, 45*(4), 904–921. doi:10.1111s/j.1475-6773.2010.01114.x

Averill, R. F., Goldfield, N., Hughes, J. S., Bonazelli, J., McCullough, E. C., Steinbeck, B. A., . . . Tang, A. M. (2003). *All Patient Refined Diagnosis Related Groups (APR-DRGs): Methodology overview. Version 20.0.* Retrieved from http://www.hcup-us.ahrq. gov/db/nation/nis/APR-DRGsV20MethodologyOverviewandBibliography.pdf

Bureau of Labor Statistics. (2008). *Occupational outlook handbook* (O*NET 29-1111-00). Retrieved from Bureau of Labor Statistics, www.bls.gov/oco

Hawthorne research. (2011). In *Encyclopædia Britannica.* Retrieved from http://www .britannica.com/EBchecked/topic/257609?Hawthorne-research

Henri Fayol. (2011). In *Encyclopædia Britannica.* Retrieved from http://www.britannica .com/EBchecked/topic/202986/Henri-Fayol

Herndon, J. H., Hwang, R., & Bozic, K. J. (2007). Healthcare technology and technology assessment. *European Spine Journal, 16*(8), 1293–1302.

HSS. (2006). *An inpatient prospective payment system overview: Diagnosis related groups.* Retrieved from Advance for Health Information Professionals website: http:// health-information.advanceweb.com/Article/An-Inpatient-Prospective-Payment-System-Overview-Diagnosis-Related-Groups.aspx

Kocakulah, M. C., Putman, T., & Vermeer, T. E. (2004). Evaluation of new technologies by hospitals and other healthcare providers: Issues to consider. *Research in Healthcare Financial Management, 9*(1), 49–56.

Kotter, J. P. (1995, March–April). Leading change: Why transformation efforts fail. *Harvard Business Review OnPoint, 1*–10.

Lookinland, S., Tiedeman, M. E., & Crosson, A. E. (2005). Nontraditional models of care delivery: Have they solved the problems? *The Journal of Nursing Administration, 35*(2), 74–80.

Malviya, A., Ramaskandhan, J., Holland, J. P., & Lingard, E. A. (2010). Metal-on-metal total hip arthroplasty. *The Journal of Bone and Joint Surgery: American Volume, 92*(7), 1675–1683.

Medicare physician payment up slightly (Again). (2011, January 30). *Orthopedic Network News*, paras. 14–15. Retrieved from http://www.orthopedicnetworknews.com/private1/jul00default.html

Pande, P. S., Neuman, R. P., & Cavanagh, R. R. (2002). *The six sigma way team fieldbook: An implementation guide for process improvement teams.* New York, NY: McGraw-Hill.

Peter F. Drucker. (2011). In *Encyclopædia Britannica.* Retrieved from http://www.britannica.com/EBchecked/topic/171933/Peter-F-Drucker

PricewaterhouseCoopers. (2005). *HealthCast 2020: Creating a sustainable future.* Retrieved from http://download.pwc.com/ie/pubs/Healthcast_2020.pdf

Proctor, J. M., Bateman, N. W., & Meurer, C. (2006, August). *IV.8: The materials management executive as a key partner in the acquisition of new technology.* Paper presented at the Association for Healthcare Resource & Materials Management's 44th Annual Conference and Exhibition, Orlando, FL.

Rao, H. (2010, October). What 17th-century pirates can teach us about job design. *US Airways*, 15–18.

Redmond, B. F., & Martin, A. L. (2011). *Need theories.* Retrieved from https://wikispaces.psu.edu/display/PSYCH484/2.+Need+Theories

Sataline, S., & Wang, S. S. (2010). Medical schools can't keep up. *The Wall Street Journal.* Retrieved from http://online.wsj.com/article/SB10001424052702304506904575180331528424238.htm

Shermer, M. (November 2008). Five fallacies of grief: Debunking psychological stages. *Scientific American.* http://www.scientificamerican.com/article.cfm?id=five-fallacies-of-grief

Simons, J. A., Irwin, D. B., & Drinnin, B. A. (1987). *Psychology: The search for understanding.* New York, NY: West.

Skorup, T. E. (2008). Evaluating new products and technology: Getting the most value for your organization. *Healthcare Financial Management, 62*(12), 96–102.

Straker, D. (2006). *Change techniques.* Retrieved from http://changingminds.org/disciplines/change_management/creating_change/creating-change.htm

Taylorism. (2011). In *Encyclopædia Britannica.* Retrieved from http://www.britannica.com/EBchecked/topic/1387100/Taylorism

Tiedeman, M. E., & Lookinland, S. (2004). Traditional models of care delivery: What have we learned? *The Journal of Nursing Administration, 34*(6), 291–297.

van den Heuvel, J., Does, R.J.M.M., & Bisgard, S. (2005). Dutch hospital implements six sigma. *Six Sigma Forum Magazine, 4*(2), 11–14.

van den Heuvel, J., Does, R.J.M.M., & Verver, J.P.S. (2005). Six sigma in healthcare: Lessons learned from a hospital. *International Journal of Six Sigma and Competitive Advantage, 1*(4), 380–388.

Van Kooy, M., & Pexton, C. (2005). Using six sigma to improve clinical quality and outcomes. *Six Sigma Healthcare.* Retrieved from http://healthcare.isixsigma.com/library/content/c030415a.asp?

Appendix A

Helpful Websites

Organization	Website	Comments
Agency for Healthcare Research and Quality	http://www.ahrq.gov	Federal agency for improving health care safety, quality, and efficiency
American Academy of Neurology	http://www.aan.com	Practice guidelines and tools
American Association of Critical-Care Nurses	http://www.aacn.org	Professional organization for critical care nurses
American Association of Heart Failure Nurses	http://aahfn.org	Education, clinical practice, and research
American Association of Neuroscience Nurses	http://www.aann.org	Professional organization for nurses
American College of Cardiology	http://www.cardiosource.org/acc	Offers clinical statements and guidelines within the field of cardiology
American Heart Association	http://www.heart.org/HEARTORG	Voluntary health agency with a mission of reducing disability and death from cardiovascular disease and stroke
American Hospital Association	http://www.aha.org	National organization representing hospitals; health care networks patients and communities
American Nurses Association	http://www.nursingworld.org	Professional organization for registered nursing
American Organization of Nurse Executives	http://www.aone.org	Membership organization of nurse executives; networking education
American Psychiatric Nurses Association	http://www.apna.org	Professional organization for psychiatric and mental health nurses
American Stroke Association	http://www.strokeassociation.org	Patient education resources

Organization	Website	Comments
Association of Perioperative Registered Nurses	http://www.aorn.org	Professional organization for operating room nurses; education resources
Center to Advance Palliative Care	http://www.capc.org	Tools and training to start and sustain a palliative care program
Centers for Disease Control and Prevention	http://www.cdc.gov	Occupational safety and health; injury prevention
Centers for Medicare and Medicaid Services	http://www.cms.gov	Regulations guidance, research education, and access to additional government resources
Current Nursing	http://www.currentnursing.com	Information and articles on management, research, education, and nursing theories
Department of Health and Human Services	http://www.hhs.gov	General information on health, regulations, and preparedness
Discover Nursing	http://www.discovernursing.com	General information for nurses, including lists of all major nursing organizations and resources
Emergency Nurses Association	http://www.ena.org	Professional organization of emergency room nurses
Health Resources and Services Administration	http://www.hrsa.gov	Division of Department of Health and Human Services (HHS); website with information for access to health care services
Healthcare Financial Management Association	http://www.hfma.org	Publications, education, and newsletters on health care finance
Home Health Nurses Association	http://www.hhna.org	Professional organization for home health and hospice nursing
Institute for Clinical Systems Improvement	http://www.icsi.org	For members only, however, offers free guidelines; order sets and sample care paths
The Joint Commission	http://www.jointcommission.org	Evaluates and accredits health care organizations
The Leapfrog Group for Patient Safety	http://www.leapfroggroup.org	Advocacy website for patient safety
Mayo Clinic	http://www.mayoclinic.com	General information and education on diseases and conditions
MedlinePlus	http://www.nlm.nih.gov/medlineplus	Health information from the National Library of Medicine

Organization	Website	Comments
National Institute of Neurological Disorders and Stroke	http://www.ninds.nih.gov	Clinical trials; guidelines for stroke treatment
National Institute of Nursing Research	http://www.ninr.nih.gov	News and research; education
National Institutes of Health	http://www.nih.gov	Information on health topics; education; additional resources; independent not-for-profit website
Nursing Center	http://www.nursingcenter.com	General information and resources for education; articles; clinical and professional topics
Regional Palliative Care Program	http://www.palliative.org	Clinical information on palliative care, including the Edmonton Symptom Assessment System (ESAS)
Substance Abuse and Mental Health Services Administration	http://www.samhsa.gov	Information on programs and publications for improving the quality and availability of substance abuse prevention, alcohol and drug addiction treatment, and mental health services
WebMD	http://www.webmd.com	General public information on health

Appendix B

VAT Toolkit

EXAMPLE OF PRODUCT EVALUATION FORM

Product Reviewed: _____ Date: _____

Manufacturer: _____ Product Number:_____

Will this replace a product currently in use? ☐ Yes ☐ No   Item Number: _____

Manufacturer: _____ Product Number: _____

Standardization Potential: ☐ Yes ☐ No   Potential annual cost savings for this product: $ _____

To Be Completed by Person Evaluating Product

Name:_____ Title: _____

Department Name: _____ Division: _____ Dept #: _____

	Yes	No	Equal to existing product	N/A
1. Easy to use?				
2. Acceptable to patient?				
3. Acceptable for procedure?				
4. Easy to store?				
5. Is the packaging label easy to read?				
6. Does the packaging open with ease?				
7. If the item is sterile, does it open without jeopardizing the sterility of the contents?				
8. Of evaluating a kit, are all the components consistently needed for the procedure?				
9. What are the advantages of this product over the one we presently use? _____				
10. What are the disadvantages of the product?				
11. Will this product improve patient outcomes? If yes, how? What are specific measurable outcome improvements? _____				
12. Would a supply of this product need to be stored in your unit?				
13. In addition to the questions above, briefly state your opinion of this product:				

(continued)

Medical Staff Review

Physician Name:_____   Title: _____

Department Name: _____   Division: _____   Dept #: _____

	Yes	No	Equal to existing product
Is this an acceptable product? If no, please explain: _____ _____			

Are there any unique circumstances where ONLY this product
  would be effective?
  If yes, please explain: _____
_____			

How does this product improve patient outcomes? _____ _____ _____			

Our Overall Review: (Please check one)
  ☐ Acceptable for use   ☐ Not acceptable for use   ☐ Additional samples required

Please return form to: _____   Dept/Division: _____

Place additional comments below:

EXAMPLE OF PRODUCT REQUEST FORM

Product Description: _____   Brand Name: _____

Manufacturer: _____   Catalog #:_____

Recommended Vendor Name/Phone #: _____

Quantity Requested: _____   Unit of Measure:_____

Instructions (Check one):

☐ **Urgent Request – Complete Section I & II.**

   ***Definitions of Urgent: (1) Life threatening, (2) Urgent/emergent surgical procedure, (3) Patient specific need (clinically indicated implant, DME), (4) Efficiencies will be impacted

☐ **Routine Request – Complete Section I & III only.**

Section I

Date: _____

Name: _____   Title:_____

Department Name / Number / Division: _____

Telephone # / Pager #: _____

Physician Requesting Review: _____

Section II – URGENT REQUEST: Processed within 2 hrs. (Must be in Purchasing Department by 1:30 pm for next day delivery)

Time submitted: _____

	Yes	No
1. Requires immediate review, no comparable product available, product anticipated to raise the standard of patient care.		
2. Will use of this product affect any other department?		
3. Is this product FDA approved?		

List: _____
    (Example: Post surgical drain that affects postoperative nursing care)

Physician Signature: _____

Department Manager Signature: _____
    (Manager may sign in Physician's absence)

(continued)

Section III	Circle One		
	Yes	No	N/A

1. Could this product replace a similar product currently in use:
    If yes, item # or manufacturer # _____
    What are the advantages? _____
    What are the disadvantages? _____			

2. Is the cost of the product greater than $100?			
3. Is the annual expenditure for this item anticipated to be greater than $1,500?			
4. Could the product potentially be used in multiple departments?			
5. Will new/additional equipment be needed to use this product?			
6. Does the product/kit contain items that are unused or not needed? If yes, explain _____			
7. Is additional staff or patient education required to use this product?			
8. Is the product invasive (enters body space) or does it come in contact with non-intact skin or mucous membranes?			
9. Will the product require a change from reusable to disposable products (or vice versa)? If yes, explain _____			
10. Is this product used as a cleaning, disinfectant, sterilization or antiseptic agent?			
11. Is the product designed to protect the patient from risk of exposure to infection? (e.g., surgical drapes , wound or IV dressings)			
12. Is the product personal protective equipment or a safety device? (e.g., needleless system, needle box)			
13. Does this product contain (circle one) PVC plastic and/or latex?			
14. Does the product use or produce a hazardous chemical?			
15. Is this product, when <u>attached</u> to patient, connected to an electrical or battery operated device?			
16. Does the vendor offer a recycling or exchange program for this product?			

Forward completed form to the Purchasing Department. All incomplete forms will be returned for completion. Call the Value Analysis Director at _____ with questions.

Requester: _____

Department Manager Signature _____   Date: _____

PURCHASING USE ONLY

☐ Approved for Purchase: PO# _____ Price each: _____ Confirmed by: _____

☐ Request forwarded to Value Analysis Director (VAD)

    Buyer's signature: _____   Date: _____

☐ Approved ☐ Not Approved   Reason: _____

    VAT Signature: _____   Date: _____

EXAMPLE OF JOB DESCRIPTION

Draft Draft Draft

Job Title: Director of Value Analysis

Job Class #: _____   **Review Date:** _____

Work Unit Name: Materials Management/Value Analysis   **Number:** _____

Department Name: Department of Finance

Signature: Department _____

Human Resources _____

**Organizational
Relationships:**   This position will receive direction from the Division Chair of Materials Management and the Physician Chair of the Supply and Services Value Analysis Committee. The individual will also work collaboratively with physicians, allied health professionals, administrators, Finance Department staff, Foundation Materials Management staff, vendors, and other individuals internal and external to XXX.

Position Overview: This position will have responsibility for achieving supply expense management initiatives and targets utilizing the value analysis process on a total annual spend in excess of $XXX million. As such, the position will direct the value analysis process to provide high quality, efficient, and cost effective products and services. This process will require the establishment and adherence to a streamlined method for standardizing and monitoring product/service selection, utilization, and costs. The incumbent will provide clinical and strategic expertise that facilitates supply expense management while continuously improving all processes that support patient care, education, and research.

Job Duties/Performance Expectations:

Job Duties	Performance Expectations Defined as Job Behaviors, Job Skills, and/or Outcomes
1. **Directs the Value Analysis Process**	a. Directs product/service introduction (internal/ external), investigation, analysis, education, conversion, issues, and tracking projected outcomes. b. Maintains a process for the continual identification and prioritization of cost containment opportunities. c. Decreases product/service expenditures by selection of the most effective and economical quality product/service based on trial and/or evaluation methods that are fact based. d. Measures, monitors, and analyzes product/ service usage and expenditures. e. Directs vendors in the value analysis process and communicates roles and expectations for business partners.

(continued)

Job Duties	Performance Expectations Defined as Job Behaviors, Job Skills, and/or Outcomes
	f. Guides project sponsors (team members) with conducting value analysis processes (e.g. procedures, work effort, information). g. Acts as project sponsor on value analysis investigations where appropriate. h. Interacts with physicians, clinicians, and allied health professionals to determine need and initiate supply/service evaluation process. i. Collaborates with evaluators and suppliers to obtain necessary products/services for evaluation as needed. j. Coordinates products/services evaluation and trials to assure the proper use of products, use of appropriate evaluation criteria, documentation of evaluation outcome, and consultation of necessary personnel (e.g. physicians, infection control, biomedical engineering). k. Ensures written summary/cost analysis and recommendation relative to evaluated product/service. l. Participates in contract negotiations with vendors. m. Manages the implementation of approved product/service conversions through collaboration with Materials Management, educational resources, suppliers and user groups as needed. n. Coordinates the resolution of any problems associated with product conversions.
2. Coordinates efforts of Supply and Services Value Analysis Committee	a. Coordinates with Division and Committee Chair to set strategy and agendas. b. Participates as a member of Foundation Value Analysis Committee and coordinates initiatives between Foundation and XX. c. Establishes/distributes agenda for meetings one week prior to meetings. d. Facilitates discussions in meetings. e. Prepares/distributes minutes of meetings at least two weeks prior to the next meeting. f. Maintains files to provide a documented reference. g. Maintains cost savings, increase, avoidance files and submits quarterly to the Supply and Services Value Analysis Committee. h. Obtains reports from team members for distribution with agenda. i. Coordinates new product requests for agenda prioritization. j. Maintains policy and procedure for the value analysis process.
3. Customer Service	a. Develops and maintains professional working relationships; utilizes networking and teambuilding skills to accomplish goals and meet customer and team needs. b. Prepares and presents timely information based upon customer requests or anticipated needs. c. Guides customers with Value Analysis Committee proposal preparation.

Job Duties	Performance Expectations Defined as Job Behaviors, Job Skills, and/or Outcomes
4. Serves as an Information Resource	a. Provides data/information related to the Value Analysis process and achieving supply expense management. b. Investigates new or alternative products/ services based on observations, product issues, excessive costs, requests from user groups, suppliers, or as assigned by the Division Chair of Materials Management or Chair of the Supply and Services Value Analysis Committee. c. Collaborates with user groups and suppliers to develop product specifications and to determine availability and potential use of standard or custom supplies. d. Collaborates with Finance colleagues in determining impact of product/service selections on revenue and accounting cycles. e. Keeps current on technology, regulatory and operational trends in the health care industry which may impact product/service utilization. f. Supplements knowledge base with available resources within and outside the organization in order to effectively accomplish various duties. g. Provides benchmarking expertise and information.
5. Manages Product Problems and Recalls, as Required	a. Coordinates collaboration between materials management, suppliers and user groups to achieve effective and efficient resolution. b. Seeks direction from legal and risk management, when appropriate. c. Maintains documentation to comply with legal/regulatory requirements and parameters established by XXX.
6. Promotes and Educates on the Value Analysis Concept	a. Acts as a resource to departments regarding the establishment of the most cost effective approach to product/service need, price, utilization and ability to support quality patient care. Recognized as an expert in value analysis. b. Develops and presents programs that will increase awareness and accountability for supply expense reduction utilizing value analysis. c. Presents program and initiative updates to division, department and institutional leaders. d. Represents XXX Clinic and participates in professional organizations and activities to establish networks and resources. e. Participates in scholarly activities; continuously improves skills and knowledge.
7. Problem Solving Ability and Objective Thinking	a. Makes decisions on emergent issues expeditiously, while considering needs of various stakeholders. b. Demonstrates strong analytical skills to perform "what if" analysis and to address the numerous issues and scenarios involved in proposed programs and processes. Gathers, researches, analyzes, and presents in an objective, non-biased "third party" manner. c. Supportive of Group Purchasing Organization contracts, Foundation initiatives and local entity strategies without losing focus of specific facility stakeholder needs.

(continued)

Job Duties	Performance Expectations Defined as Job Behaviors, Job Skills, and/or Outcomes
8. Administrative/ Leadership	a. Leads institutional and/or department/division teams and projects that contribute to the on-going improvement of work processes, procedures, systems, quality and customer service. b. Leads and actively participates in cross divisional/departmental and institutional teams, councils, and workgroups.

Education/Experience/Job Skills:

Requires a Bachelor's degree in Nursing with a minimum of 7 years in a clinical/progressively more responsible role in a diverse and operationally complex health care environment. Masters in Business Administration, Health Science, or related discipline preferred.

- Experience in cost containment and expense management activities.
- Proven management skills, including program planning and development, project management, and performance and quality management.
- Demonstrated analytical experience with a knowledge of financial and accounting concepts.
- Excellent interpersonal relationship skills and the ability to drive consensus.
- Computer competency–Microsoft suite–(Word, Excel, PowerPoint) required. Knowledge of Access desirable.
- Strong communication skills which will encompass both oral and written including the ability to give presentations to physicians, clinicians, and administrators.
- Demonstrated problem-resolution skills.
- Understands inter-workings of supply chain activities.
- Ability to interact and manage relationships with vendors.

EXAMPLE OF AGENDA AND MEETING NOTES

Heading:

Subject: Surgical Services VAT	
Date/Time:	
Location:	
Teleconference Information: xxx-xxx-xxxx	

Agenda/Notes:

Meeting called by:	
Invited:	
Attended:	
Agenda	**Notes/Minutes**
Next Steps:	

Action Items:

Action Items Generated from Meeting						
AI #	Action Item	Date Assigned	Date Due	Owner	Date Completed	Notes

EXAMPLE OF VAT TEAM: SURGICAL SERVICES CHARTER

Approved by: _____   **Date approved:** _____
Executive Sponsor

Approved by: _____   **Date approved:** _____
Initiative Lead

1) Initiative Management Team

Role	(Name & Phone)	(Name & Phone)
Sponsor		
Team Lead	TBD	

2) Team Roster

Name	Hospital/Department	Title	Phone
	Corporate Distribution Center (CDC)	Director or Representative	
	Materials Management Surgical Services	Manager or Product Representatives	
	Surgical Services	Team Leader or Staff/GYN	
	Surgical Services	OR Staff/Urology Tech	
	Surgical Services	Staff Nurse Urology	
	Surgical Services	Tech GYN	
	Surgical Services	Staff Nurse GYN	
	C- Sterile Processing	Staff	
	Surgical Services	OR Tech	
	Maternal-Child Nursing	Staff Nurse Labor & Delivery	
	Cardiology	Staff Nurse Cardiology	
	Surgical Services	Staff Nurse Surgery	
	See attached detailed list of Participants.		

3) Objectives & Target

Total Targeted dollars savings for Team:
Annualized Savings Range: $1.6 mil – $2.2 mil

Objectives (Expected Improvements)
1. Increase product and vendor standardization and utilization to decrease Surgery supply cost;
2. Improve GPO contract compliance to reduce surgery supply costs
3. Improve the process of inventory management and control, focusing on critical item management and demand planning;
4. Streamline processes for product selection, utilization, and cost management;
5. Standardize operating policies and procedures and improve controls, reduce cycle time, and eliminate redundancy and variability;
6. Reduce inventory to increase efficiency, improve service outcomes, and achieve one-time costs savings;
7. Integrate supply chain processes across the System, utilizing technology and best practices to maximize outcomes and resource utilization in both labor and facility management;
8. Implement an Enterprise-wide in-service education and communication program for surgical services supply chain changes;
9. Establish outcomes measurement and reporting process

4) Scope
Boundaries (e.g., scope, authority) 1. The Surgical Services (SS) Work Group or Value Analysis workgroup (VAW) will be responsible for realizing the targeted (perioperative) surgical services supply chain savings as a part of the overall Supply Chain initiative. 2. The SS VAW will be responsible for identifying and implementing cost savings opportunities for the Perioperative Services Departments. 3. The SS VAW will work in conjunction with the overall Value Analysis Oversight Committee (VAOC) to coordinate activities, which may bridge other HM Value Analysis workgroup. 4. The SS VAW is responsible for communicating activities related to the decisions made by the team to the (VAOC), Perioperative Staff, and Surgeons. 5. The SS VAW is responsible for identifying and minimizing barriers to implementing cost savings opportunities.
Assumptions 1. Annualized savings opportunities will be strongly contingent on effective, integrated technology. 2. Hospital will provide accurate and timely data from the Purchasing, Information Systems, Materials Management, and Finance departments. 3. Hospital's educational resources will be responsible for coordinating future in-service training to ensure staff and surgeon knowledge related to SS VAW supply chain process and utilization, policy and procedure changes and practices. In-service training should be coordinated with vendors when appropriate. 4. HM Perioperative and other staff will be available, as needed, to actively participate in SS VAW meetings and activities.
Key Implementation Issues and Risks Inability to access accurate data, lack of integrated systems and core materials management functionality; 1. Ability of staff to support accelerating change and maintain awareness of the business imperative; 2. Information systems ability to report complete and accurate cost/utilization data; 3. Ability of the organization to quickly react to necessary changes in structure and process for implementing identified opportunities.

5) Key Milestones: Work Steps, Deliverables, Performance Measures to be Achieved	
Milestone	**Targeted Completion Date (Mo/Day/Yr)**
1. Establish VAW composition, members, gain commitment	July 16, 2010
2. Conduct kickoff meeting	August 20, 2010
3. Identify and integrate current projects into VAW	August 27, 2010
4. Develop communication plan	August 27, 2010
5. Identify standardization, utilization reduction, and cost savings opportunities	September 3, 2010
6. Collect product usage information	September 3, 2010
7. Identify non-standardized product pricing across system	September 3, 2010
8. Identify opportunities to transfer excess inventory across system	September 3, 2010
9. Develop implementation plan	September 17, 2010
10. Communicate recommendations to the VA Oversight Committee	September 24, 2010

(continued)

11. Present recommendations to the Physician Advisory Group	September 24, 2010
12. Develop policy and procedures (as needed)	September 24, 2010
13. Redesign and implement processes (as needed)	September 24, 2010
14. Develop education and training plans	September 24, 2010
15. Implement recommended changes in products, policies, procedures and processes across the System	December 31, 2010
16. Develop tracking and documentation tools	September 24, 2010
17. Track supply chain measures	On-going – IRW's

6) Initial Hit list: (In Part) Separate Document for HM VA Work Groups
1. Endoscopy supplies, trocars, instrumentation
2. Custom packs and kits
3. Inventory management (par level management & use of slow moving owned items (intraocular lenses, ortho implants)
4. Surgical draping practices
5. Intraocular lenses (opthalmics)
6. Skin stapling devices
7. C/V – valves, grafts
8. Specialty gloves
9. Orthopedic – orthopedic implants and hardware & software
10. Other implants
11. Surgical instruments (scissors, graspers, needle drivers, dissectors)
12. Sutures, consolidation, standardization
13. Urological/Cardiovascular stents, guidewires, catheters
14. Minor equipment
15. Wearing and personal protective equipment apparel
16. Reprocessing of single use and open and unused items

7) Deliverables:	
1. Workgroup charter and detailed Initiative work Plans	July 30, 2010
2. Status reports	Ongoing
3. Targeted opportunities List	Ongoing
4. Surgical services supply management process, policies, procedures	September 24, 2010
5. Completed IRWs	

8) Areas of Overlap		
Initiative/VAW	**Other Projects**	**Implication(s) for Your Work**
1. Logistics/ distribution 2. Sourcing/ procurement	Procurement, distribution, sourcing, Inventory management	Integration and consolidation; Processes (Supply, Storage and acquisition), Information/Data Access, Contract Management
3. Pharmacy	Procurement, distribution, sourcing, Inventory management	Drug utilization, system-wide Formulary, pharmacy inventory Management
4. Interventional/ diagnostic VAWs	Procurement, distribution, sourcing, Inventory management	Product standardization, Impact on Utilization
5. Radiology VAWs	Procurement, distribution, sourcing, Inventory management	Product standardization, Impact on Utilization
6. Other VAW as identified	Procurement, distribution, sourcing, Inventory management	Product standardization, Impact on Utilization
7. MMIS technology	Integration and access to data related to supply usage, pricing	Integration and consolidation; Processes, Information/Data Access, Contract Management
8. Gen Med-Surg VA Work Groups	Procurement, distribution, sourcing, Inventory management	Product standardization, Impact on Utilization

EXAMPLE OF VAT—STATUS REPORT

January 26, 2009

Key Resources	
Project Sponsorship:	
VAT Team:	

Project Description			
Key Milestones / Deliverables	**Start Date DD/MM/YY**	**Finish Date DD/MM/YY**	**Status**
Submit data request	21/12/06	21/12/06	Complete
Kick-off meeting	08/01/09	08/01/09	Complete
Confirm project scope, timing, and deliverables	08/01/09		In Process
Implementation milestones agreed	08/01/09	06/02/09	In Process
Receive data from Data Request	10/01/09		In Process
Analyse data	11/01/09	31/01/09	In Process
Conduct interviews	10/01/09	31/01/09	In Process
Evaluate e-Requisitioning project	19/01/09		In Process
Map procurement processes	22/01/09	31/01/09	In Process
Develop strategy to address storage/inventory levels	22/01/09		In Process
Develop implementation plans regarding product standardisation and utilisation	10/01/09		In Process
Engage Consultants and Nurses			
Discover and implement "quick wins"	22/01/09		In Process

Status Highlights January R A G					
Executive sponsorship	G	Interviews	G	Implementation plans	G
Schedule	G	Data collection and analysis	G	Scope	G
Facility tours	G				

Major Accomplishments in this month–

- Reviewed drafts of overall product flow and product top-up process maps
- Reviewed draft of purchasing process map
- Reviewed draft of ICD and pacemaker analysis with
- Began review of product flows
- Began draft of Procurement process straw model
- Began overall standardization and rationalization analysis

Major activities and plans for next month–

- Meet to review CSSD product flow
- Review Theatre product flow for Day Surgery
- Review draft of Procurement process straw model and recommendations with Alistair
- Interview and tour TSSU
- Complete quantification of ICD and pacemaker scenarios opportunities
- Continue Pharmacy analysis
- Continue validation of available data

Other key issues :

-

Decisions for Steering Group:

-

G	**On-target** (No-issue)		**A**	**At risk** (Minor issues)	**R**	**Behind target** (Issues require immediate attention)

Index

NOTE: Page numbers followed by "f" indicate figures and "t" indicate tables.

Accommodate, conflict management type, 203
Acquisition, 48
Adjusted average daily census (ADJ ADC), 8t
Adjusted patient days (APD), 94
Admissions and discharges, 25f
Advertising roles, in supply costs, 53
Agency nurses, 6
All-Patient DRGs (AP-DRGs), 105
  hierarchy, 110
  major complications and comorbidities in, 110
  pediatric and other modifications, 110–111
All-Patient Refined DRGs (APR-DRGs), 105
  development of, 111–112
Amerinet (GPO), 70
Amortization, 93
Annual budget, 89–102
  budget *versus* actual analysis, 97, 97t
  creation of, 95–97
  department, 96f
Average daily census (ADC), 8t, 14, 20, 136, 144

Balance sheets, 90
  consolidated, 91f
Bed assignment, 20, 155–156, 158
Bed assignment dashboard, 161f
Bed placement, 136
Bedded units, 20
Benchmarking reports, 146
Black Belts (BBs), in Six Sigma, 152, 182

Budget, 3, 4, 7, 18, 21, 24, 45–46, 50–51, 53–54, 69, 72, 74–77, 87, 89–90, 94–95, 97, 103, 115, 125, 149
Bulk distribution, 49–50

Capacity optimization, 125
Capacity to demand, 20
Capital equipment expenditures, 76–78
  budget and approval processes, 77–78
Care delivery techniques, 125–150
Care pathways and roadmaps, 128
Case management, five performance parameters, 134
Case management subgroup, 133–134
Case manager assistant, 136
Case managers, 135
Case mix complexity, 107
Case mix index (CMI), 51–52
Centers for Medicare and Medicaid Services (CMS), 21, 54, 103–113, 165
Change management, 198–203
  psychology behind, 198–199
  theories and models, 199–203
Chief financial officer (CFO), 89
Commonwealth Health Corporation (CHC), Six Sigma and, 151
Communication, 187–194
  with physicians, 204–206
Communication charter, sample, 192–193f
Complications and comorbidities (CCs), 110
Compromise, 203
Conflict management, 203
  accommodate, 203
  avoidance, 203

Conflict management (cont.)
  collaborate, 203
  compromise, 203
  dominate, 203
Conflict resolution, 203–204
Consumerism, in supply costs, 53
Contemporary nursing models, 17–23
Continuing education, component of
      motivation, 186–187
Continuous Quality Improvement (CQI), 154
Contract language, 117
Coronary artery bypass graph pathway, 147f
Cost center (CC), 94
Cost effectiveness, 69–82
Cost modeling, 55–56
Current state bed assignment process flow,
      157f–159f
Cushion ratio, 93

Daily census, 8t
Daily staffing plan, 7, 14t
Damaged goods, 50
Days in accounts receivable (AR), 93
Department budget reviews, 51–53
Depreciation, 93
Diagnosis-related groups (DRGs)
  classifications for atypical information,
      108–109
  patient classification system, 107–110
  revisions for Medicare, 109–110
  role in patient care reimbursement, 105–108
Direct care hours, 8t
Direct costs, 94
Dismissal, 36–37
Distribution, 49
  methods, 49–50
DMAIC (Define, Measure, Analyze,
      Improve, and Control), 152–154
Draft products communication agenda,
      189–190f
Drucker, Peter, 179, 212
Drucker's management by objectives,
      179, 212
Drug diversion, 208
Drug Enforcement Administration (DEA)
      license, 208

eAuctions, 76
ECRI Institute, 186–187
Episodes of care (EOC), 123

eSourcing, 76
Evidence-based medicine (EBM), 126, 174
Expensed upon receipt, 79

Facilitated sessions, 209–215
Fastest Finger Quiz, 213
Fayol, Henri, 178
Fayolism, 178
Financial analysis, 55–56
Fixed costs, 94
Fixed hours, 8t
Flex staffing model, 18–20
  applying to labor and productivity,
      23–30
  float pools in, 28–29
  staffing coordinator, 27–28
  use of sitters in, 29–30
Float pools, 6
  role in flex staffing model, 28–29
Food and Drug Administration, 47
Forecasting demand, 24
Full-time equivalents (FTEs), 14
Functional care model, 16–17
Future state day of surgery process flow, 142f
Future state PAT process flow, 141f
Future state scheduling, 140f
  preassessment process flow and, 143f

General ledgers, 51
Generally accepted accounting principles
      (GAAP), 90
Generated productivity report, sample, 40t
Graphic organizer, 183
Green Belts (GBs), in Six Sigma, 152
Grief stages, 198–199
Ground-up budget process, 77
Group purchasing organization (GPO),
      43, 69–72
  contracts, 70–71
  intermediate agreement management
      scenario, 72t
  multivendor, 71t
  optimized agreement scenario, 72t
  unmanaged agreement scenario, 71t
Guardian tasks, 32

Hawthorne effect, 178–179
Health care costs, advertising and
      marketing in, 53

Health care finance, 87–102
    common terms, 90–91
    operating budgets, 95
    purchasing considerations, 98–100
    strategic planning, 94–95
Health maintenance organization (HMO),
    115–118
Health system pharmacy service, 206
HealthTrust (GPO), 70
Hierarchy of needs, 198
Hospital unit clerk (HUC), 15
Hostile management, 181
Hours allocated from other departments, 7
Hours per patient day (HPPD), 14
Human resources (HR), 14, 31
    issues, 177

Income (profit and loss) statements, 90
Incorrect use of supplies, 50
Indirect costs, 94
Individual motivation, 186
Individual rate of acceptance, 198
Inpatient Prospective Payment System
    (IPPS), 104
Inpatients, 9t
Insulation management, 180
Intangible asset, 93
Integrated delivery network (IDN), 70
Integrated model, 18
Internal rate of return (IRR), 55
Inventory, 93
Inventory form, 100f
Inventory management, 78–82
    classification, 79
    clinical inventories, 79f
    conducting physical inventory, 80
    supply chain metrics/definitions,
        80–81
    understanding purchase orders,
        81–82

Joint Operations Committee (JOC), 116
Just-in-time (JIT) distribution, 50

Kotter, John, 201–202
Kotter's Eight-Step Change Model,
    201–202
Kübler-Ross, Elisabeth, 198–199
Kübler-Ross Grief Cycle, 198–199

Labor
    applying flex staffing model, 23–30
    productivity and, 3–4
Labor costs, 1
Leadership skills, 175
    case study, 217
Length of stay (LOS), 126, 131f
    case study, 165–174
Lewin, Kurt, 199–200
Lewin's Change Model, 199–201, 200f
Licensed practical nurse (LPNs), 14
Long-distance management, 180
Low unit of measure (LUM) distribution, 50

Major Diagnostic Categories (MDCs),
    105–106, 128
    cost per case by, 132f
    length of stay by, 131f
Managed care, 115–119
    contract language, 117
    contracting, 116
    reimbursement, 116
Management by objectives, 179
Management style, 177–180
    troublesome styles, 180–181
Managing change, conflicts, and
    relationships, 197–216
Managing resources, 24
Maslow, Abraham, 198
Maslow's Hierarchy, 180f, 198
Master Black Belts (MBBs), in Six Sigma, 152
Materials management information system
    (MMIS), 48, 57f, 78
Mayo, Elton, 178–179
Mayo Clinic, 186
MedAssets (GPO), 70
Medicare and Medicaid. *see* Centers for
    Medicare and Medicaid Services (CMS)
Medication administration records, 207
Memo, sample, 191f
Midnight census, 9t
Min/max levels (PAR), 49
Mind map, 183
Missed charges, 50
Monthly key performance indicators, 162f
Motivation
    individual, 186
    strategies to keep tasks on track, 182–183
    strategies to promote, 182
Motivational dynamics, 183–186
MUDA (wasteful activity), 152

Need for intervention, in case mix
complexity, 107
Net cash flow, 94
Net present value (NPV), 55
New product request process, 59f
New technology
Medicare and Medicaid reimbursement, 55
overuse and responsible use, 55
purchasing, 54
New Technology Assessment Committee
(NTAC), 53–54, 75
Nonbedded units, 20
Nonclinical model, 18
Nonlabor expenses, 45–46, 46t
Nonpartnered clinical model, 18
Nonrelevant costs, 54
Notes receivable (NR), 93
Novation (GPO), 70
Nurse extender model, 18
Nurse Manager, 1, 3–7, 11, 13, 24, 26, 28,
33–34, 49–51, 77–78, 187, 197–198,
204–205
productivity measurement, 3–5
workload volume control, 5
Nurse–patient ratio, 9t
Nurse ratios
advent of, 4
mandatory in California hospitals, 5t
Nursing assistant (NA), 15

Operating budgets, 95
prior period results, 95
Operating margin, 94
Operational improvements subgroups, in
patient throughput, 138
Opportunity costs, 54
Ordering process, 98
Outpatients, 9t
Overtime, 6, 7

Paid FTTEs, 9t
Paid hours, 9t
Partnership clinical model, 18
Patient care 2000 model, 18, 19
Patient care reimbursement, 103–120
DRGs in, 105–108
managed care contracts, 115–119
Patient care technicians (PCTs), 17
Patient classification, 107
Patient classification system, 22–23t

Patient days, 9t
Patient process-flow mapping, 126–128
day of surgery, 127f, 129f, 130f
Patient Protection and Affordability Care
Act (PPACA) (2012), 21
Patient safety, pharmacy relationships and,
207
Patient service partner model, 19
Patient throughput
bed placement, 136
components, 138f
physician component to, 136
questions, 137f
tracking and monitoring, 136
using process maps, 128–149
Patients per bedside nurse, 9t
Performance documentation and reviews,
33–35
Performance improvement plans (PIP),
35–36
Perpetual inventory, 79
Personal management skills, 177–195
Pharmacy relationships and communication,
206–209
medication administration records, 207
nurse education, 208–209
nursing leadership expectations, 207
patient safety, 207
state and federal regulatory compliance,
208
Physical inventory form, 100f
Physician advisor (PA), 134–135
Physician component, to patient throughput,
136
Physician relationships and communication,
204–206
Preadmission testing, 139f
Preferred provider organization (PPO),
115–118
Premier (GPO), 70
Prepaid expenses (prepaids), 93
Primary care nursing model, 15
Product acquisition report (PAR), 49
Product management, approach to, 60f
Productive hours, 10t
Productivity
applying flex staffing model, 23–30
common terminology, 7, 8–10t
labor relationship to, 3–4
measures, 1–11
Professionally advanced care team
(ProACT), 18

Profit margin, 94
Prognosis, in case mix complexity, 107
Program managers, 134
Project charter, 156t
Proposed "new" bed assignment process
      flow, 160f
PTO percentage, 10t
Purchase orders, 81, 98, 99f
Purchasing
   annual, 89–102
   considerations from the finance side,
      98–100
   new technology, 55

Recruiting, 31–33
   defining required skills, 31–33
Red Cross Hospital, the Netherlands, Six
      Sigma and, 151–152
Refreezing, Lewin's change model, 201
Registered nurse (RN), 14
Relevant costs, 54
Repressed management, 180
Resource intensity, in case mix complexity,
      107
Resource management, 123, 125–128
   approach and methodology, 132–149
   elements of, 126
Return on investment (ROI), 93
Revenue growth, 94
Risk of mortality, in case mix complexity,
      107

Sample communication charter, 192–193f
Sample memo, 191f
Scientific management, 178
Selection, 47–48
Severity of illness
   in case mix complexity, 107
   each secondary diagnosis, 113
   process of determining, 113–115
   subclass for patient, 113–115
Shrinkage, 50
Sitters, in flex staffing model, 29–30
Six Sigma, 151–163, 182–183
   applying to improving health care
      outcomes, 154–159
   five steps, 153t
   use in health care, 151–154
Skill alignment, 146
SMART objectives, 179, 212

Social workers, 135
Staffing coordinator, role shift, 26–28
Staffing models, 13–30
Staffing plans, 7–11
Staffing tools, 13–23
Star tasks, 32
STAT distribution, 50
State and federal regulatory compliance,
      pharmacy relationships and, 208
Statement of cash flows, 90
Sticking and Cycling, Lewin's change model,
      201
Strategic planning, health care finance,
      94–95
Strategic planning subgroup, 133, 133f
Subaccount, 94
Supply chain, 45–68
   acquisition, 48
   cost analysis, 52f
   distribution, 49
   distribution of expenses at facility level,
      47f
   links, 46–47
   managing the budget, 51–53
   selection, 47–48
   spending, 46
   utilization, 50–51
Supply chain contracting, 72–76
   clinician and physician involvement,
      73–74
   effecting contracting, 76
   initiating contracts, 74–75
   negotiating contracts, 73
   new technology assessment committee
      (NTAC), 75
   obtaining capital equipment online, 76
   precontract considerations, 73
   process subgroups, 148
Supply chain metrics/definitions, 80–81
Supply costs, 53–55

Target WHPPD, 10t
Task matrix, 214–215
Tax Equity and Fiscal Responsibility Act,
      1982, 105
Taylor, Frederick Winslow, scientific
      management, 178
Taylorism, 178
Team, definition, 183
Team motivation and dynamics, 181–187
Team nursing model, 17

Terminology, 7, 8–10t
Throughput, 123, 125–126, 128, 131, 133, 136–138, 151, 165
Time lines, 146–147
Time management, 194–195
Title 22 statutes, California, 4, 5t
Top-down budget process, 77
Total patient care model, 16
Total Quality Management (TQM), 154
Tracking and monitoring subgroup, 149
Transition/change, Lewin's change model, 200
Traveling nurses, 6
Treatment difficulty, in case mix complexity, 107
Trending volume, 24

Unfreezing, Lewin's change model, 200
Uniform Hospital Discharge Data Sets (UHDDS), 104
Units of service, 3
Unlicensed assistant personnel (UAPs), 17
Utilization, 50–51

Value analysis teams (VAT), 43, 56–68
  composition, 56–58
  decisions in urgent care, 58

measuring value and efficiency, 58
NTACs and, 75
role of team members, 56
roles and working relationships, 62–66
start-up checklist, 66–67t
structure, 57f
team toolkit, 61–68
Variable costs, 94
Variance report, 92f
VAT Toolkit, 225–239
Vendor standardization, physician buy-in, 83–86
Volume of work, 5

Waste, 50
  damaged goods, 50
  missed charges, 50
  incorrect use of supplies, 50
  shrinkage, 50
Work plan template, 212t
Worked care hours, 3
Worked FTTEs, 10t
Worked hours, 10t
Worked hours per patient day (WHPPD), 7, 10t

Yellow Belts (YBs), in Six Sigma, 152